THE FOUNDATIONS OF YOUR PRIVATE PRACTICE
Volume One: The Complete Guide to Starting and Developing a Successful Private Practice

Through the years
from Michael
to
Grandpa

The Foundations of Your Private Practice

Volume One
The Complete Guide to Starting and Developing A Successful Private Practice

MICHAEL I. GOLD, Ph.D.

with

Colette McDougall

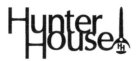

For further information contact:
Hunter House Inc., Publishers
P.O. Box 2914
Alameda, CA 94501-0914

The authors are grateful for permission received to reprint from the following:
"Guidelines for the Client Entering Group Therapy," by Ann Spadone Jacobson, Ph.D.,
Psychologist; "Client's Bill of Rights" from *The California Therapist*, the publication of
the California Association of Marriage and Family Therapists, Nov/Dec 1989, used
with permission; "Ethical Principles of Psychologists" © 1994 by the American
Psychological Association. Reprinted (or adapted) by permission; "Preamble," in The
Principles of Medical Ethics With Annotations Especially Applicable to Psychiatry.
Washington DC, American Psychiatric Association, 1992, p. 2. Copyright © 1992
American Psychiatric Association; Antioch CA 1994 the Atlanta Revision of the Los
Angeles Suicide Potentiality Rating Scale, reprinted with permission of Family Service
of Los Angeles/Suicide Prevention Center; "Advertising: A Legal and Ethical
Perspective" by Richard S. Leslie, in *The California Therapist*, 2(3) May/June 1990,
used with permission of the author; "Selling Your Private Practice: Ten Provocative
Questions" by Sherri Ferris, M.S., in *The California Therapist*, 4(1) Jan/Feb 1992, used
with permission of the author; the curriculum vitae of Dr. Richard Marsh,
used with permission.

Library of Congress Cataloging-in-Publication Data

The foundations of your private practice.
p.   cm.
Includes bibliographic references and index.
Contents: v. 1. The building of your private / by Michael I. Gold with Colette
McDougall—v. 2. the complete book of clinical forms for an effective private practice
/ by Michael I. Gold with Phyllis A. Galbraith, Jean Yingling.
ISBN 0-89793-124-6 (v. 1 : hardcover): $29.95—ISBN 0-89793-125-4 (v. 2 : hardcover):
$74.95—ISBN (invalid) 0-89793-126-2 (forms): $50.00
1. Psychiatry—Practice. 2. Psychiatry—Practice—Forms. I. Gold, Michael I.
[DNLM: 1. Practice Management, Medical. 2. Psychotherapy. W 80 F771 1993]
RC465.5F68   1993
6616.89'0068—dc20
DNLM/DLC
for Library of Congress   93–12015

Manufactured in the United States of America
9   8   7   6   5   4   3   2   1   First edition

Project Credits

Project managers: Lisa E. Lee (editorial) Paul J. Frindt (production)
Cover designs by Tamra Goris Graphics and Jil Weil Designs
Book design by *Qalagraphia*
Copyeditors: Kate McKinley, Mali Apple, Janja Lalich
Proofreaders: Susan Burckhard, Theo B. Crawford
Production Assistance: María Jesús Aguiló Pérez
Marketing: Corrine M. Sahli
Customer Support: Sharon R. A. Olson, James Rachogan
Fulfillment: A & A Quality Shipping Services
Publisher: Kiran S. Rana
Set in Palatino and Goudy Sans by 847 Communications, Alameda, CA
Printed by Publishers Press, Salt Lake City

Ordering

Individuals may order additional copies of this book or the forms packages using the order form at the end of the book. Hunter House books are available at special discounts for sales promotions, organizations, premiums, fundraising, and for educational use. For details please contact:

Special Sales Department
Hunter House Inc., Publishers
P.O. Box 2914
Alameda, CA 94501-0914
Phone: (510) 865-5282   Fax: (510) 865-4295

Trade bookstores in the U.S. and Canada please contact:

Publishers Group West
4065 Hollis Street, Box 8843
Emeryville CA 94608
Phone: (800) 788-3123 Fax: (510) 658-1834

Table of Contents

Important Notice

The material in this book is intended to provide a review of information regarding setting up a private psychotherapy practice. Every effort has been made to provide useful and dependable information. The contents of this book have been carefully reviewed by experts in the field. However, professional therapists have differing opinions and ways of approaching the practice of therapy, therefore the information presented herein should be regarded as the expertise of the authors. Also, specific rules and regulations may vary from state to state, so check with your local agencies.

The publisher, authors, editors, and reviewers cannot be held responsible for any error, omission, or dated material. The authors and publisher assume no responsibility for any outcome of the use of any of these procedures in setting up a private practice.

If you have a question concerning your own practice, or about the legal appropriateness or application of the procedures described in this book, consult your attorney.

Although many state and national agencies and associations have helped to provide information and resources for this book, the appearance of materials and/or the inclusion of information does not represent any agency or association approval of the contents of this book.

Acknowledgments

I would like to thank the many people that helped make this two-volume publication a reality. Thank you to Ted Pedersen; Emil Soorani, M.D.; Vera David, Ph.D.; Wyler Greene, Ph.D.; Harold Foster, M.A.; Harvey Mindess, Ph.D.; Mary Proteau; Richard Marsh, Ph.D.; Bob Martinez; Mali Apple, Janja Lalich and Kate McKinley; the State of California Department of Consumer Affairs and its agencies; the American Psychiatric Association; the Associations of Marriage and Family Therapists; the dozens of civil servants in local, county, and state agencies; and to the tireless people at Hunter House, from publisher Kiran Rana, production manager, Paul Frindt, and editor Lisa Lee, to assistant to the publisher Corrine Sahli; and finally, to my friend and colleague, John Ranyard.

Thank you.

Michael I. Gold
Hermosa Beach CA
January 1994

Foreword

Dr. Michael Gold is an astute clinician and teacher. He is also a mix of seemingly opposite characteristics: hard-working and self-indulgent, flamboyant yet methodical as an instructor, outspoken in conversation yet canny in therapeutic feedback. Just a regular, tormented, fun-loving man. A once-in-a-lifetime original and a true professional success.

The Foundations of Your Private Practice contains a bounty of practical advice to mental health workers and an introduction to a pragmatic philosophy of life—because establishing a successful private practice requires a good dose of both. His practical advice, the nuts and bolts of business, is spelled out clearly and succinctly and covers everything from selecting a location to terminating a practice. The philosophy, which is more often alluded to than stated outright, draws on Dr. Gold's existential outlook—the inspiration and ultimately the force behind his therapy—and touches every topic.

Read this book and take it to heart. It is the next best thing to knowing Dr. Gold personally or taking one of his courses. His book will alternately guide and challenge the reader in developing a practice and doing effective, profitable therapy.

As the former Director of the Graduate Psychology Program at Antioch University, I can attest that hundreds of students applauded Dr. Gold's teaching excellence every year. As his colleague for ten years or more, I can say that he brings both a wealth of information and an irreverent, enlivening spirit into the classroom.

And, as the friend he once described as "casting light where there is no darkness," I can return the compliment by telling you that this book contains more information than you will ever want to absorb about the business and practice of psychotherapy.

Harvey Mindess, Ph.D.
Professor Emeritus, Antioch University

Introduction

This book was created to help you open and run your private practice as a profitable business. You may use this book as a blueprint to set up a new practice, or just incorporate some of the ideas into your existing practice.

As both a clinician and teacher, I am sharing knowledge that is not merely theoretical, but that has been extensively tested in my own and others' practices. Everything in this book comes from more than 25 years of training and practice.

Many books offer valuable practical advice on how to open and run a private practice. However, they often tend to focus on how to make lots of money. But there is much more than profit to a successful and satisfying private practice: the personal satisfaction and ethical aspects; our relationship to the changing society in which we live; and the needs of our clients, which grow and evolve as they do. Consequently, nothing in this book is here simply because it is a good idea—though it may be that—it has all proved to really work.

Throughout the book I refer to a set of forms first published about 1985 in California. These forms have since been updated to fit the needs of clinicians in other states, and are now a complete package of forms for the behavioral science practitioner. They are discussed in detail in Volume Two of *The Foundations of Your Private Practice* (the book), and are also available as a separate package. For information on ordering Volume Two and the package of forms, please see the back of the book.

It is not necessary, however, to use these forms to benefit from this book. Other companies sell clinical and business forms, and you may already have forms that were designed to suit to your specialty. This book is intended to help you build a more satisfying and profitable private practice, regardless of which forms you use.

Throughout this work, Ms. McDougall, my consultant clinicians, my editors, and I have kept in mind that we are addressing you: an educated, clinically trained professional. We have tried always to keep in mind that you are the doctor.

1

At the same time, we have worked to make this text viable and to save you hundreds of hours—so that you will be able to devote most of your time to your clients, instead of reinventing the wheel of setting up and maintaining a private practice. We wish you great success and satisfaction in your practice.

Michael I. Gold, Ph.D.

1

The Ethics of Making Money

As an instructor in a graduate psychology program, I have found that 25% to 50% of my students will try to start their own private practice. However, only about 5% to 10% of those who complete their degrees and receive their licenses will retain private practice as their primary source of income. Some will keep limited practices, sharing office space and seeing three to six clients a week. Others will end up working for Employee Assistance Programs or other mental health programs. Still others will leave the field of psychology altogether.

I believe that clinicians in private practice sometimes fail not through lack of clinical competence, but from a deficiency of entrepreneurial skills and a failure to understand that they are running a business as well as serving in a helping profession.

Many clinicians and others who work in the mental health field are reluctant or guilty about making money in their chosen profession, especially early in their practice. This may be because they feel uneasy about "profiting" from the suffering of others, or because in our profession it is often difficult to say when healing has occurred and what the real agent of healing has been. It may be because they are often part of, and directly affected by, the healing process and derive considerable personal value from it. All of these hesitations, however noble, stem from a misunderstanding of the role of money in the therapist-client relationship.

To understand the role of money in this relationship more clearly, we need to begin with a discussion of Abraham Maslow's hierarchy of needs as it relates to the economic, emotional, and social functions of being a private clinician. This relationship bridges the gap between the academic clinician and the professional practitioner.

Maslow's Hierarchy of Needs

When addressing the issue of human needs, it seems appropriate to use the extensive body of work of Dr. Maslow. His hierarchy of needs addresses, in a generalized format, ideas that we must to reassess continuously—not only in our clients' lives but in our own, as clinicians. We as therapists need to address Maslow's hierarchy of needs, or we may have difficulty helping our clients to do so.

As every practitioner knows, Maslow's hierarchy of needs is a pyramid. The idea is that all humans wish to self-actualize: to make real, or actual, the life they wish to lead; to be all that they can be.

To achieve self-actualization, we must first pay attention to our physiological needs, which are located at the bottom of Maslow's pyramid—we must be fed, clothed, and housed. Once these needs are satisfied, we must fulfill our security needs, while continuing to meet the physiological needs. Next, we must have some degree of social satisfaction and, finally, some kind of ego satisfaction—a sense of personal accomplishment. Only then can we attain self-actualization.

Maslow found that addressing these needs contributes to people's happiness and self-realization. Maslow stated that a person who ignored his or her physiological and security needs would have difficulty fulfilling the social and ego needs.

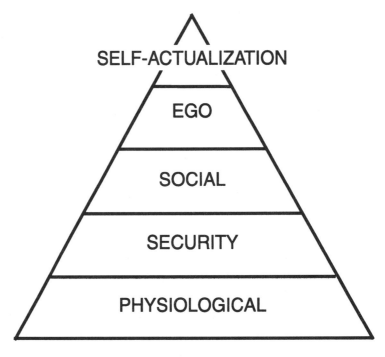

Maslow's Hierarchy

Our business, as therapists, is to help people actualize their well-being; if we are not actualizing our own well-being, through not taking care of our physiological and security needs, we may well hamper the delivery of our services. This is why therapists who don't pay attention to the economic and entrepreneurial aspects of private practice are often not successful.

If you don't take care of your physiological and security needs, you will have difficulty fulfilling your social and ego needs. An economically sound and secure psychotherapist displays a nondesperate attitude and can focus on the practice of therapy. This, in turn, enables the psychotherapist's clients to make the most of therapy, to meet their basic needs.

I am a more efficient psychotherapist today than I was 25 years ago because I have fulfilled my physiological and security needs. This does not mean that I charge more than my service is worth. Therapists engaged in the delivery of psychotherapeutic services should charge an appropriate fee, which maintains self-respect. Therapists who neglect the issue of economics and the business aspects of private practice may not survive in their profession.

Money Is Not a Dirty Word

Most therapists enter the psychology field because of a need to help people. Many psychotherapists are codependent helpers.

Codependents can be defined as caring people who overextend themselves. We often view codependents as neglectful of their own needs. It is as if codependents do not know what their personal needs are or how to meet them. They are unable to receive nurturing, and they participate in relationships that lack reciprocity.

Codependents are also often uninformed about basic economics. It is important for the therapist, as a potential codependent, to remember that *money* is not a dirty word, but instead view it as a basic form of nurturing. Money does not buy happiness, but it does buy food, shelter, and other physiological necessities, leaving people free to consider choices and options in other areas.

Clinicians must take stock of their own levels of functioning, as is done by the diagnostic procedures in the DSM. It is all too easy for clinicians to focus on their clients' issues in relation to Axis IV (psychosocial stressors) and Axis V (levels of functioning) and never take the time to examine their own stressors and levels of functioning. Economic issues seem to be among the leading causes of intrapersonal and interpersonal stress, so it is important to address these issues up front. While people in the helping professions typically are not economically driven, we all use economic status, to different degrees, to define our own worth, even though we know it is not a true measure. This does not mean that a careful evaluation of our economic needs should be neglected. Without that, we may fail to meet our most basic needs and, thus, be unable to address our higher goals.

The Myth of Getting What You Pay For

You do not always get what you pay for! In many ways, we are more energized, wondrous, and exploratory as interns charging no fee than we are later on as experienced therapists charging over $100 per session. As interns, we do not yet know that we can't "cure" some clients and, as a result, we often do.

"Putting on the robe of the therapist" means bringing your own process of self-actualization to your work. When you are able to meet your own needs, you will be able to convey a message of faith to your clients. After having achieved a measure of self-actualization, you can pass that and other experiences on to your clients.

This book is an attempt to assist you in getting your own needs met so that you can be fully present to care for and respect your clients. Caring without reciprocity is irresponsible, and that irresponsibility creates a climate of dysfunction. If we are irresponsible to ourselves, we cannot be responsible to our clients. Unfortunately, many people who receive their licenses are not responsible to themselves and end up not practicing because of it.

Therapists' and Clients' Responsibilities to Each Other

Psychotherapeutic healing in the behavioral sciences typically requires mutual responsibility. This involves therapist and client informing one another of the initial boundaries and conditions of the relationship and informing one another when there is a perceived necessity to change it. We have an economic relationship with our clients that is governed by laws and ethics. We also have a psychological relationship with our clients, which forms the basis of transference and countertransference.

Throughout the course of your career, there will be times when it will seem as if you and your client are drowning together. Picture your office as a swimming pool. You and your client must dive into issues in order to move toward resolution. As a clinician, it is your responsibility to keep one hand always on the side of the pool—to maintain a steady grip on the situation.

This means that you are responsible for keeping your client informed of the economic side of your relationship as well as the psychological. Do not leave your client guessing about your fees; they are an essential part of the boundaries determining your relationship. As with other boundaries in the therapeutic relationship, do not hesitate to discuss them with your client if either of you feels the need for a change.

Setting Your Fees

Here's the best piece of advice I have ever received: Never charge what you are worth; charge what you need to support the life you choose to live.

Set your fees based on what you need. This is a service profession: you are paid a fee for performing a service. When starting your practice, you may feel your services are not worth much. In this case, set your fee based on the fee that you wish you could charge.

Set your fees in line with the going rate charged by other clinicians, with similar credentials, who are practicing in your general location, and present that fee at the outset. If you wish to see a client at $5 an hour, that remains your prerogative. Your *fee* is still $75 an hour. This is an extremely important concept to convey to your clientele. Presenting your fee in this way to the "$5-an-hour clients" reminds them that they are getting a good deal. It will also encourage them to refer clients to you who can afford your desired fee of $75 a session.

Any fee negotiated below your customary fee should be subject to change every six months. Fees may need to increase due to sudden inflationary trends or changes in the status of your private practice for a multitude of reasons, e.g., you become famous overnight for having published a book. Whenever possible ask your current clientele, depending on their ability to pay, to increase their payment. Negotiate with any new clients at the increased rate.

A typical fee increase per year is 10% or $10.00. Inform your clients what they can expect. We all respond better to increases in expenses when we are warned in advance. You may tell them that if they are unable to pay the increase, you will continue to see them at the former rate until it becomes an economic hardship for you. A standard practice is to charge existing clients the percentage increase (e.g., 10%), and to quote new clients the higher, standard fee.

If a few of your clients are unable or unwilling to pay your new fees, it is your responsibility to refer them to a clinician who charges a fee they can afford and who has similar credentials. This is not only ethically sound, it is good business sense. The clients you refer will remember that your willingness to help them extended to your helping them find a therapist they could afford.

Setting your fee to get the lifestyle you want is another way of creating reciprocity in your life. Reciprocity is not a simple exchange based on "tit for tat," but an exchange of comparable worth. In such an exchange people give and receive with balance. If you equate your price to worth, you may miss the point.

Even in a system that provides for socialized medicine—which by default may well be the wave of the future—Maslow's hierarchy of needs must still be addressed. In that same vein, as private practitioners, I believe you need to address your own basic attitudes and beliefs—and own them or discard them based on the productivity they bring your life.

Nothing in Your Training Prepares You for Private Practice

When I was training as a psychotherapist, my supervisor, my therapist, and my mentor were all the same person. Because I attended graduate school, was in therapy and under supervision, was educated in the workings of private practice, and had treated clients, by the time I received my license, I was fully acquainted with the minutiae of running a private practice. For most students today, such an ideal arrangement is no longer possible.

The separation of research from clinical practice in our field has deepened so that practical, clinical concerns are often not addressed until an intern is actually in practice. Additionally, it seems to me, state boards and professional associations are, unconsciously or consciously, alienating students of psychology from the realities of private practice in order to protect the economic interests of professionals who are already licensed. Some of the ways that state boards may discourage private practitioners are by continuously changing requirements; by refusing to accept interns' hours of training; by holding "requirement and licensing provision meetings" without allowing interns, practitioners, and state association members to attend; and by designing state examinations that are ambiguous, deceptive, and do not truly test the clinical competency of future practitioners.

I unequivocally believe that the training and licensing procedures in place today tend to disable competent and caring healers and to enable the more obsessive and noncaring, narcissistically focused professionals in our society. As a clinician, you need to discover your own expertise and to know your strengths—and your vulnerabilities. I hope that this book's attention to detail will empower you to manage your practice as the kind of environment in which you can care for and respect yourself and your clients.

Lifestyle Should Dictate Work Style

Many of us allow social organizations—families, schools, governments—to dictate to us the lifestyle we should lead. Since we are in the business of helping people actualize their individual needs, it is necessary to actualize our own needs. But first we must discover those needs and make our goals accordingly.

Having your own goals will help you to become your own person. The more concrete your goals, the more directly you will be able to act upon and understand them.

There is a saying: "Do you know how to make God laugh? Tell him your plans." At any time in our lives, our path may change because "someone makes us an offer we can't refuse. " Nevertheless, having goals can have a profound impact on our lives.

When formulating goals it is often helpful to write them down so as to be able to physically contemplate them. I use the following exercises with my clients and in seminars and classes. In doing these exercises people often recognize for the first time the presence or absence of their goals and, as a result, the meaning they want to give to their lives.

The most important and powerful part of these exercises is the writing. The process of putting thoughts on paper makes them more clear.

The first exercise is intended both for you and your clients. In the exercise you will examine your wishes. Your wishes reflect what you want in your life and, more specifically, how you want to live your life.

Exercise 1. My Ultimate Life

This is an exercise in which you set down your dream life—no holds barred, no limits other than your heart's desire. What would you do to make a day perfectly yours? Write down your thoughts. Then, change them if you want to.

My Ultimate Day The format your writing takes is not as important as the act itself. If you feel more comfortable with a schedule or an essay or even just a series of notes, put your day in that form.

By envisioning your desires and committing them to paper, you have taken the first step toward reaching your goals. Although we may not accomplish some of our goals, we develop a sense of well-being when we have a direction and purpose. The function of goal-setting is to explore how you feel about your needs and channel them into an "Ultimate Life."

My Ultimate Week For your Ultimate Week, imagine what you would do with seven days entirely at your disposal. Would you live them all the same as your Ultimate Day? Would you spend more time on some activities than on others? How would you break up your days? Don't forget to include time for relaxing. The only limit is your imagination.

My Ultimate Month Now expand your Ultimate Day and Ultimate Week into an Ultimate Month. You can repeat your Ultimate Week, change it around, take a vacation; do what you want.

My Ultimate Year Given that you are living your Ultimate Day, Ultimate Week, and Ultimate Month, how would you build your Ultimate Year? Since there are no limits, you may go anywhere you wish, do anything you desire, and spend time with whoever you wish at any time you wish for as long as you like. Once you have established goals and a plan, you know what to say yes or no to. Hold on to your dream and work toward it.

Many of us live our lives without any notion of where we are going. If we do have a notion about our purpose, we often lack a plan. This is equally true of clients entering psychotherapy and of professionals in the psychology field.

Defining our goals gives us a chance to take a concrete look at our dreams. There is an enormous difference between wishing something, wanting something, and having the willingness to get it.

My Ultimate Life

My Day:

My Week:

My Month:

My Year:

Exercise 2. My Want Ad

In this second exercise, you will complete a mock-up of a full-page ad to run on the back page of your city's largest newspaper. (See the example on page 13.) In the top two sections, describe yourself when you are functioning at your best and when you are functioning at your worst. In the "Who I Am" section, list all of your positive qualities and your shortcomings. In the "What I Want" section, describe in detail what you are in search of; for example, you might list all the qualities you would like in a partner. Life has a way of giving us exactly what we ask for. So, the better job you do at telling the truth about yourself in the "Who I Am" section and at being explicit about your needs in the "What I Want" section, the more likely you are to get what you want.

Designing your want ad will aid you in putting down on paper your wants, needs, and goals so that you can see them in black and white. By keeping these goals in sight, you can include and exclude people and circumstances as needed to aid you in your self-actualization.

Although at times it may seem that some of your goals will never be reached, doing these exercises can help you learn to say no. By setting down your goals clearly, as in these exercises, you can learn to prioritize according to your goals, instead of according to what is important to those around you or what is "supposed" to be important. Learning to say no points us more clearly to the yesses of life.

These exercises have helped me channel my energies to find my path, as well as enabling me to find the kinds of people I wish to include in my life. They may help you find your path as well.

At My Worst!

My Want Ad

At My Best!

Who I Am:

What I Want:

2

The Economics
of Private Practice

This chapter discusses how to estimate initial opening costs, ongoing expenses, and income for the private practitioner. Formulas are introduced for quick calculations of accounts receivable income and accounts payable expenditures. It also discusses the entire economic structure of a private practice—as well as economic projections.

Managing Your Money

Even though you may be a private practitioner operating a cottage-level industry (i.e., out of your home or rented office space, or in a part-time practice), it is my recommendation that you place the money you earn as a clinician in a separate account from any other income. Apart from the billing record and running-total bookkeeping, a business bank account serves as a running tabulation of the money flow in and out of your practice. Having a separate account will save you many hours in preparing tax returns. You will be able to tell exactly how much money came in from your practice as well as how much it costs to run the practice. Since the account is separate, it will be easier not to spend your household expense money on supplies for the office, or income from your practice on dry cleaning.

Furthermore, a business bank account is extremely helpful as an economic assessment of your practice, especially for clinicians with other vocational business concerns. This system allows you to determine whether you need to increase your billing for your practice to become self-sufficient. You may find that you need to close an office because it is not producing enough revenue. It's okay to learn that something is not working. Not to know whether something is working is not so smart.

Tax Laws and the IRS

Let's talk about billing no-no's.

Any money over $600 paid to you by an insurance company will be reported to the federal government. (Check with your accountant for changes in this tax law after 1993.) Until 1978, many clinicians made false claims to insurance companies, padding their charges. These clinicians were actually charging their clients half the billed amount. Needless to say, these clinicians lost their licenses or, in some cases, were sent to prison. The tax law was then changed. Clinicians are now taxed on the amount billed, rather than the amount collected.

For example, if I were to bill an insurance company $100 for a session, and the insurance company then pays 50% of that balance, I need to collect the other 50%, or $50, from my client. If I am audited, an insurance company will presume I have collected the $50. Let's suppose the client did not pay me. I must have a small-claims judgment against the client to present to the IRS for that $50, or the IRS can assume that I collected the money and did not report it.

Your tax liability is based on what you tell the insurance company you were going to collect. If you are audited, your tax records must show the full fee. If you did not collect the money, the IRS will expect that you attempted to collect it by filing a small-claims judgment. This is how the IRS operates with private practitioners. As a rule of thumb, accountants have told me that the IRS also presumes that 80% of your practice is billed through insurance companies and 20% is cash-based.

It is a good idea to figure out your tax bracket well in advance and make a habit of setting aside a percentage of your income for taxes. Remember, as your income increases, so do your taxes, and you may need to re-figure your tax bracket throughout the year. One way to make this easier is to pay your taxes on a quarterly basis and thus avoid the April squeeze.

Rental Costs

The average size of a consultation room is about 250 square feet (about 12½ feet by 20 feet). The waiting room can be anywhere from 40 to 110 square feet. Sometimes you can alter the configuration of an office depending on your needs (e.g., by moving a wall or installing a partition). In most U.S. metropolitan areas, you can expect to pay a minimum monthly rent of $1.50 to $2.00 per square foot for an office. You will also be charged for what are referred to as common areas. Common areas include walkways, restrooms, and so forth. Generally this will be a flat surcharge figured into your rent.

For example, an office of around 350 square feet rented full-time with a one- to five-year lease in a reasonable area of Los Angeles will cost approximately $700 to $750 a month. Divided by five for a typical five-day work week, this comes to $150 per "day-month." This day-month method of calculating rent will let you know how much money to charge or pay when subletting. Under this system, if you lease your office to a clinician who wants to use all the Mondays or all the Tuesdays in a month, you should charge one-fifth of your monthly rent. Sublet contracts should never be for less than one year, so you would then multiply the day-month figure by twelve and contract with the clinician for that amount.

It is also possible to calculate office rent by the hour. However, if you are subletting an office space, the lack of commitment implied in hourly renting as opposed to daily or monthly renting can limit your practice and unconsciously lead you to procrastinate marketing your services. If you don't feel you have a real stake in the office, you may not be as eager to bring in clients who will help pay for it. So, when subletting, I recommend you do it by the day, not by the hour.

The distinction between subletting a space to someone else versus subletting another clinician's office is essentially a matter of control and responsibility. You may have less control over available hours of office use when subletting from someone else. You may find that as a master tenant who sublets space, you have more economic responsibility in the maintenance of your office. Whatever arrangement you choose, it is extremely important to determine the exact schedule of usage by you and the other clinician, and to explore the opportunities for expanding or limiting the time available to each of you. In addition, if you are sharing an office with more than one clinician on any given day, allow at least two hours as a transition time between one clinician and the other (this is addressed further in Chapter 7).

Malpractice and Other Insurance

One of the questions you must answer when starting a practice is whether you wish to carry malpractice insurance. This is often overlooked in estimating the cost of a practice. Malpractice insurance is a clinician's protection against lawsuits regarding professional conduct. Almost all policies also contain public liability insurance, which protects the clinician against suits relating to "accidents" (such as falling down stairs) that might arise in and around your office environment. Although most landlords carry public liability insurance, a clinician who decides to carry insurance should include public liability coverage, because unfortunately, in most public liability suits, the clinician will be named as a defendant. For a nonmedical psychotherapist, a policy covering both professional and public liability will generally cost between $250 and $1,200 a year, depending on the amount of coverage (typically, between $1 million and $3 million). Check with your local and state associations for the best deals on malpractice insurance.

When considering malpractice insurance, the issue of becoming a "target defendant" comes into play. Simply put, if you carry insurance, an attorney is more likely to take a case against you than if you do not carry insurance. Many professionals are now posting signs in their waiting rooms informing their clientele that they are not covered by insurance. The other side of the issue is that someone may have a paranoid personality disorder with a tendency to be "suit happy" (litigious), in which case you will need the protection of insurance.

Malpractice insurance is, in some ways, attorney insurance. Because the insurance company must handle all claims against its insured, it protects you against "nuisance suits," which can be costly in both time and money. Business and professions attorneys cost up to $350 an hour. Having insurance frees clinicians from the fear of paying sizable attorney's fees.

Fire and theft insurance will add to your insurance costs. To obtain fire and theft insurance, you will be required to show that your building meets special codes. Check with your local fire department to get their standards for fire-safe buildings and for locks.

Always pay careful attention to the clauses and exclusions on a policy. Sometimes they exclude everything for which you can be sued! Contact your state and national professional organizations for insurance company recommendations.

Expenses: How Much Will This Cost?

You will have noticed that in all the discussions of cost so far, I have given a range of possible costs. How much it will *actually* cost to open the door to see your first client depends on a number of factors: where you decide to practice, the sort of office you decide to have, whether you rent or sublet, what kind of insurance you want, etc.

In our culture, offices are often perceived as reflecting the way clinicians feel about the worth of their services. Since your office will generally be the first thing a client sees of you, it is worth the cost to have a presentable office. This can be done economically with good planning and taste.

Practicing out of your home may be less expensive than having a separate office, but it can be disruptive to your personal life. It may also place you and your family at risk from clients who act out against their therapists. Consider the cost of an office the price you pay to protect your privacy.

Using a mid-range projection, assuming you are opening an office in a metropolitan area and taking into consideration such costs as lease deposits, furniture, phone installation, business licenses and fees, insurance, lighting, stationery, and water coolers, your initial cash outlay will be between $4,000 and $7,000.

Once you have made this initial outlay, however, you must still have money to cover monthly operating costs. For example, for a sole practitioner seeing individuals, families, and small groups and renting a full office, monthly costs including rent, office and waiting-room supplies, and phone bills will run $1,000 to $1,500 per month. You must set enough cash aside to cover these costs for several months, until you have enough clients to cover them.

These expenses can be drastically lowered if you are a beginning or part-time practitioner who is sharing initial costs. By renting space from an established practitioner, or setting up a new a practice with several colleagues, you could pay $125 to $150 rent for one day a week. With phone bills of $50 to $100, and supplies and membership fee costs of $50 to $100, your monthly costs can be as low as $350 to $400.

Most of your decisions regarding setting up your office will be based on your financial situation. Initially, I recommend that you rent space from an established practitioner so that your costs are low and you can focus whatever capital you have on acquiring clients.

Income to Expense Ratios

I highly recommend that at the beginning of your career you try to keep an income-to-expense ratio of 6 to 1. In other words, for every $100 you earn in fees, your monthly operating expenses should not be above $15–18. To begin with, though, it may be hard to stay above a ratio of 4 to 1. If your monthly operating costs are $300 to $400, you need to make $1800 to $2400 a month. If you have six clients a week paying $50 a session, that is $300 a week or $1200 a month. So, you may need to raise your fees—which may be difficult, especially when the economy is depressed—or lower your costs. Making accurate projections of income is discussed further in the next section.

When I first began my practice, I rented an office from a clinician on an hour-by-hour basis. This enabled me to have an office and to begin my practice without spending a lot of money up front for furniture, phones, rent, and such. As my practice grew, I rented by the day; within a year I was able to rent by the month. Over the years, I have come to realize that most clients do not care about a fancy office. A convenient, central location, ample and well-lit parking, and the physical comforts of appropriate room temperature, user-friendly furniture, and considerate but practical lighting in the session room are much more important that high-priced trimmings. Like New York, Los Angeles rentals are extremely expensive. Yet, whether I was subletting from another clinician or other clinicians were subletting from me, I have always been able to find comfortable offices in good locations, and I have generally been able to maintain an income-to-expense ratio of 6 to 1. By keeping expenses down, I have been able to survive more difficult economic times. In our field, fancy offices do not necessarily translate to good practitioners or high-paying clients. Keep this in mind when searching for your first office or when reevaluating your current situation.

The "Client Count"

Therapists play a game with one another called the "client count." This is where you ask another therapist the question, "How many clients do you have?" In playing, you discover that another clinician may have 37 clients while you may only have 6, and you begin to wonder what you are doing wrong.

This is the economic equivalent of adolescents comparing penis or breast size. The act of comparing can in itself be destructive and is only rarely informative. Unless you know the clinician well, he or she will either boast about the number of clients he has or give you a thousand reasons why his practice is low.

The client count is one of the myths of psychotherapeutic practice. The success of your practice cannot be measured by how many clients you have. What is relevant is how many collectible, billable hours your practice generates each week.

If I am asked how many clients I have, I could rightfully say 60. My answer then raises another question, "How can you do 60 hours of psychotherapy a week?" I could either lie and say that I like long hours or tell the truth and admit that many of my clients have sessions only twice a month. Furthermore, I sometimes have as many as eight or nine clients attending one session.

In other words, the "number" of clients is irrelevant.

Making Income Projections and Staying Out of Debt

When I try to estimate income from my practice for a year I use a concept I call the "year-hour." Let me explain: most clinicians see a regular client at the same time on the same day each week. So, if I see Client X on Tuesdays from 3:00 to 4:00 P.M., then over a year of 52 weeks I will see her 52 times. Client X's Tuesday time-slot is one year-hour. If I charge her $50 per 50-minute session then that year-hour is worth $2,600. Multiply that by the number of hours you can work in a week and you get wonderful numbers that can have the dollar signs dancing in your head. In reality, however, there are many factors that limit those numbers.

To start with, you need a vacation. Let's say you take a two-week vacation every year. So now your year-hour is worth $2500 not $2600. The next factor to consider is how many regular, year-round clients you can get, or how many hours a week you can fill with long-term and short-term clients. If you are new to private practice this next bit of information may shock you: the average full-time private practice is 15 hours per week. As a beginning practitioner, after one year, if you have done the groundwork to build up your practice, you can expect to be seeing clients 7 to 12 hours a week. At an average of 10 hours per week times $2500 per year-hour your annual income will be $25,000.

This is why most clinicians have a second occupation. Many of them teach. Others work part-time with social service agencies and private companies, or provide personnel services, do research, write, review, etc. The ones with the gift of eloquence go out on the lecture circuit and do trainings, workshops, and seminars.

But wait, there's more. Here is another rule of thumb for projecting your income that comes from my clinical experience: you should use 40 sessions per year per full-time client in your projections to estimate your income accurately, not 50. Let's go back to Client X, who is paying $50 for one 50-minute session per week. If she comes once a week and pays $50 per session, the total income from her over the 52 weeks in a year minus a 2-week vacation should be $2,500. But in reality, your 2 weeks of vacation might not coincide with her vacation. Add to that time off due to illness (yours or hers) and appointments not kept because of a time change (e.g., daylight-saving time), the illness of a family member, traffic jams, and the thousands of activities that can legitimately prevent her from making it to therapy every week, and you end up, not with 50 sessions per year, but closer to 40.

This will leave you an additional 10 to 12 hours for scheduling clients who may need to see you more than once a week because of a crisis in their lives. It also will leave you time to catch up on records, bookkeeping tasks, or report writing. Finally, it gives you time to lie down and take a nap.

Another way to view this is to say that you need a 25% client to fill those 10 session-hours that are left open by Client X in one year, or that you need 1.25 clients for a year-hour. Except that you really need 2 clients for a year hour: one full-time client and one 25% client.

When I make income projections, I multiply my session fee by 40 and then multiply that by the number of my regular clients to estimate my baseline annual income. For example, if I have 10 true-blue clients who are dedicated to their psychotherapy, the total yearly income from them will be 10 times $50 times 40 sessions, which equals $20,000. In order to fill those 10 hours for the entire year, though, I will need at least another 10 part-time clients.

This brings me to what I call the client-to-session ratio, which is the number of clients you need to fill one billable year-hour. If you are just beginning your practice, review at the end of your first year how many hours you were in session and how many clients it took to fill those hours. If you have been practicing for years, look at your records for the past several years to find the same information. One of the ways of staying out of debt is by maintaining a profitable client-to-session ratio.

From talking with colleagues, especially those beginning a clinical practice, I have found that at the beginning of a practice it takes as many as 7 to 12 clients to fill one year-hour. This is especially true if you decide to have a goal-oriented, cognitive-behavioral practice. This style of practice tends to create more client turnover than the more traditional forms of psychotherapy.

Established clinicians may only need four, or even as few as two, clients to fill one year-hour. What this implies is that if you want to work 20 sessions per week, you will need to anticipate providing treatment to at least 140 different clients at the start of your career. That is why it is extremely important to develop a large client base.

This brings up another important aspect of developing a practice, and that is keeping track of where your clients are coming from. I ask my private practice interns and the people who attend my seminars to calculate what percentage of their client base was referred to them, and what their major sources of referral are. Some psychotherapy clients wish to "keep you to themselves," and will refer few, if any, clients. Others, though they may see you only for a brief period of time, can be excellent referral sources. Some clients have provided me directly or indirectly with 200 new clients, while others who covet our relationship rarely, if ever, refer people to me.

The ability to predict year-hour utilization and client requirements allows clinicians who have been in practice for 10 to 20 years to accurately estimate their income for the following year. And those who maintain a large and varied client base are better able to survive lulls in their practice, barring natural or economic disasters beyond their control.

Billing

Among the first tasks in your clinical training were the establishment of a fee schedule and signing an agreement to that effect. It is recommended that you continue this procedure in your private practice. Many clinicians post a sign in their office, stating in effect, *The Doctor Will Be Delighted To Discuss Fees Any Time.*

In general, clients pay at the end of each session. Some clients may wish to be billed once a month. Depending on the client, you may or may not want to accommodate this request. Also be aware that, based on your diagnosis of a client, you may need to insist on payment up front.

I recommend that your fee schedule be stated in a contract form and be discussed during the first session. Make it clear to your clients whether you expect invoices to be paid upon receipt or within a certain time. For example, you may wish to be paid within 10 working days of the client's receipt of the invoices, and will start charging interest after 60 days. Also be sure to discuss your policy openly with prospective clients during the first session.

Insurance Companies

If you do not accept insurance checks as payment for services, your bookkeeping system need not be complex. Your billing statement can indicate for insurance companies to remit money directly to the client, while the client pays you. Periodically, you may encounter an insurance company that cannot pay the client because of state law. In this instance, ask the client to pay you, accept payment from the insurance company, and pass it on to the client.

There are several ways of accepting payment from insurance companies and passing it on to the client. With your client's permission, you may choose to include the insurance company's payment as part of payment for services rendered or payment for services to be rendered. Another way to repay your client is to sign insurance reimbursements directly over to them. Lastly, you can deposit insurance reimbursements in your business checking account and write a check to the client from that account.

Before delivering reports or filling out forms for various insurance companies, get the appropriate clearances from your client for a release of confidential information (see page 70). Some insurance companies will have these releases on their forms, so you will not need to use a separate form. You may also wish to contact the person or persons who will be reviewing the forms or reports to get an understanding of what will help the insurance company make a clear decision. This allows you to focus on the clinical information necessary to aid both the client and the provider so that the clients may continue to receive necessary services without economic hardship.

The procedure for billing an insurance company is simple. When a client brings you the insurance form, write on it, "See attached form"; then use instead the form you normally use. Staple the two forms together, have the client fill out the appropriate portion of the insurance form, and send it all to the insurance company. (It is a good idea to keep a copy of anything you send to an insurance company. Most practitioners today have access to a copy machine, and personal copiers can be purchased for as little as $300. You may also want to print as NCR forms those that leave the office, such as forms for the release of confidential information.) Sometimes insurance companies will send you a letter asking if the diagnosis is work-related. You can respond to them either in writing or by telephone.

When billing an insurance company, you must list your federal tax identification number or your social security number. Some forms of billing do not require your social security number, so before you have it pre-printed on your forms, consider whether you feel this violates your privacy.

Your fee must be the same whether or not you are billing an insurance company. To do otherwise is unethical. You can, however, have a sliding scale based on other factors. Rather than only considering income, it is a good idea to look at such particulars as, "Does she have children?" "Does he live alone?" "Is she recovering from an economic crisis?" The answers to these questions often make a big difference in a client's ability to pay.

Billing Statements I and II

Billing statements should be sent on a fixed, prearranged schedule (e.g., every month or every three months). They can be sent directly to the client, attached to the provider's insurance form, and/or sent directly to the insurance provider. Insurance companies generally do not want clinicians to submit a separate bill for each session.

Billing Statements I and II, on pages 25 and 26, are designed to give you flexibility in creating the clinical and aesthetic look you wish. Some clinicians prefer to use predesignated procedure numbers and CPT codes (as in Statement II), while others would rather use a format that allows for more sessions per billing statement (as in Statement I).

When preparing these forms always be sure to date them.

Have your client check with the insurance agent or call the company to find out if you need a referring physician or preauthorization to treat the client. You must do this before submitting a billing statement. Not all insurance companies require this, but some still do, so be sure to check.

On my billing statement, I include several pieces of information. If a client has been referred, I list the person and the date of referral. I indicate which professional services were provided and itemize these services with dates. I list the diagnostic number using the DSM-III-R.

I always reference the diagnosis that I consider to be the least harmful to the client while still being clinically accurate. I am sad to report that certain diagnoses can unwarrantedly affect the rest of a client's life. Diagnoses such as schizophrenia, bipolar illness, depressive illness, and psychological factors affecting physical condition can lead to a client

Date: **STATEMENT**

To:

Name of Insured:

Address:

City: **State:**   **Zip:**

Name of Client: **Relationship to Insured:**

Referring Physician: **Date:**

The following professional services were provided to the above-named client as itemized, and on the dates listed below, for the diagnosis of:

DATE	SERVICE RENDERED		CHARGE
	Procedure Code	Description	

Clinician's Signature: **TOTAL:**

Soc. Sec. No./Fed. ID No.

State License Number:

Form FPP-19-1/1-rev2/94 ©1994 GMS. Limited permission to photocopy only. For orders call (510) 865-5282, fax (510) 865-4295.

Date:	STATEMENT		

Name of Insured:	DIAGNOSIS	
Address:	Axis I	
	Axis II	
	Axis III	
Name of Client:	Axis IV	
	Axis V(a)	
Relationship to Insured:	Axis V(b)	

Date	Service Rendered		Total Fee	Balance
	* Procedure	Description		
		Balance Now Due		

* No.	Procedure	CPT
1	Individual 50 minutes	90844
2	Individual 25 minutes	90843
3	Family/Conjoint	90847
4	Multiple-Family	90849
5	Group	90853
6	Report Preparation	90889
7	Diagnostic Interview	90801
8	Testing, with Report	90830
9	Telephone Consultation	98920

Clinician's Signature:

SSN or Federal ID Number.

State License No.

being refused medical and disability insurance in the future, and in some cases, certain diagnoses can disqualify a client from a job or a security clearance. Just as we have a responsibility to insure the safety of our clients and to keep other people from harm, we also have a responsibility not to cause greater harm.

I do not suggest that you falsify or lie on an insurance document or forensic report. However, do be aware of the potential repercussions on your clients' future. When your professional ethics require you to use these sensitive diagnoses, let your client know the implications of their billing reports. This knowledge is part of their basic civil right.

Unfortunately, insurance companies often seem to relate to psychological diagnoses in an uninformed and inappropriate way. Most insurance companies are now using utilization review boards (URBs) to serve as middle men to "allow" for treatment. Utilization review boards seem to accept only certain diagnoses for specific, limited periods of time, using medical models and medicine as the acceptable forms of treatment. Stay current and in contact with your utilization review boards, as they may prove to be a diversionary tactic that insurance companies use in order not to cover necessary services. Tell your state professional associations about the utilization review process as you experience it.

Utilization review boards, if unopposed by our profession, could be one of the leading tactics insurance companies will use to replace the private practitioner with the corporate practitioner. This is an extremely dangerous and potentially disastrous situation for clients who need psychological help that does not conform to a preconceived and incorrect treatment model devised by insurance companies and economically prejudiced psychological consultants.

The Superbill

The Superbill is a great time saver because it includes Current Procedural Terminology (CPT) codes and diagnostic coding, and it is available in the NCR (no carbon required) triplicate format. The Superbill should be used on a fixed schedule over the course of therapy.

Depending on the size of your practice, there may not be a great deal of difference between using Billing Statements I or II or the Superbill. Billing Statements I and II require more written information, since both diagnostic and procedural codes must be entered by the clinician. They also require photocopying for you to keep a copy for your records. If you try them both out in your practice for about a year, you should get a good idea of which is better for you and your practice in terms of

SUPERBILL

DSM-III-R DIAGNOSIS

DEVELOPMENTAL DISORDERS	DISSOCIATIVE DISORDERS
DSM-III-R:	DSM-III-R:
ORGANIC MENTAL DISORDERS	SEXUAL DISORDERS
DSM-III-R:	DSM-III-R:
SUBSTANCE USE DISORDER	SLEEP DISORDERS
DSM-III-R:	DSM-III-R:
SCHIZOPHRENIA	FACTITIOUS DISORDERS
DSM-III-R:	DSM-III-R:
DELUSIONAL DISORDER	IMPULSE CONTROL DISORDERS
DSM-III-R:	DSM-III-R:
PSYCHOTIC DISORDERS	ADJUSTMENT DISORDERS
DSM-III-R:	DSM-III-R:
MOOD DISORDERS	PSY FACTORS AFFECTING PHYS COND
DSM-III-R:	DSM-III-R:
ANXIETY DISORDERS	PERSONALITY DISORDERS
DSM-III-R:	DSM-III-R:
SOMATOFORM DISORDERS	V CODES
DSM-III-R:	DSM-III-R:

	DATE OF SERVICE	CPT CODE	CHARGES
1.			
2.			
3.			
4.			
5.			
6.			
7.			
8.			
9.			
10.			
TOTAL			

POLICY HOLDER	INSURANCE CARRIER	POLICY NUMBER
POLICY HOLDER'S SSN	ADDRESS	CITY STATE ZIP
CLIENT'S NAME Circle M F	RELATIONSHIP TO POLICY HOLDER	CLIENT'S BIRTHDATE
REFERRED BY	DATE SYMPTOM FIRST OCCURRED	LOCATION SERVICES RENDERED OFFICE OTHER

AUTHORIZATION TO PROVIDE INFORMATION TO INSURANCE CARRIER:
I HEREBY AUTHORIZE THE RELEASE OF ANY INFORMATION ACQUIRED IN THE COURSE OF MY EXAMINATION AND TREATMENT.

SIGNATURE   DATE

AUTHORIZATION TO ASSIGN BENEFITS TO PROVIDER:
I CERTIFY THAT THE SERVICES LISTED HAVE BEEN RECEIVED AND I AUTHORIZE PAYMENT TO BE MADE DIRECTLY TO SAID CLINICIAN.

SIGNATURE   DATE

PROCEDURE CODES	90844 45–50 MINUTES
HOSPITAL CARE	90847 FAMILY PSYCHOTHERAPY
90200 BRIEF HIST AND EXAM	90849 MULT FAM GRP PSYCHOTHERAPY
90215 INTERMEDIATE HIST AND EXAM	90853 GROUP PSYCHOTHERAPY
90220 COMPREHENSIVE HIST AND EXAM	90870 ECT: SINGLE SEIZURE
90240 EACH DAY, BRIEF SERVICES	90871 MULT SEIZURES PER DAY
90250 LIMITED SERVICES	90880 HYPNOTHERAPY
90260 INTERMEDIATE SERVICES	90882 ENVIRONMENTAL INTERVENTION
90270 EXTENDED SERVICES	90887 INTERPRET OF EXAM RESULTS
90280 COMPREHENSIVE SERVICES	90889 UNLISTED PROCEDURE
90292 HOSPITAL DISCHARGE	*BIOFEEDBACK*
THERAPEUTIC INJECTIONS	90900 BIOFEEDBACK TRAINING
90782 INJECTION OF MEDICATION	90904 REG OF BLOOD PRESSURE
SPECIFY:	90906 REG OF SKIN TEMP
90784 INTRAVENOUS	90908 BY EEG APPLICATION
INTERVIEW PROCEDURES	**MEDICAL PROCEDURE CODES**
90801 DIAGNOSTIC INTERVIEW EXAM	*OFFICE VISITS*
90825 EVALUATION RECS OR REPORTS	90020 INIT COMPREHENSIVE EVAL
90830 PSYCHOLOGICAL TESTING	90060 INTERMEDIATE VISIT
90831 TELEPHONE CONSULTATION	90070 EXTENDED VISIT
90835 NARCOSYNTHESIS	*HOSPITAL CONSULTATIONS*
THERAPEUTIC PROCEDURES	90620 INITIAL, COMPREHENSIVE
90841 INDIV. PSYCHOTHERAPY; UNSPEC	90630 INITIAL, COMPLEX
90843 20–30 MINUTES	90643 FOLLOW-UP

TODAY'S DATE

PROVIDER'S SIGNATURE

TYPE OF LICENSE, STATE LICENSE NUMBER

PROVIDER'S FEDERAL TAX ID OR SSN

cost and time. It is worth the initial investment to try both forms and will help you develop a record-keeping and billing style to suit your specific needs.

The most important thing to consider when deciding between billing statements and the Superbill is your personal preference and the way you keep track of your economic records. The Superbill may be more efficient and expedient, but the habit of preparing a regular billing statement is still preferred by many clinicians.

You may find that the cost of processing forms for insurance companies is not worth the money you get from it. In addition, the time it takes to fill out the simplest of superbills can leave you far less time to do the work you are trained to do. Insurance company hotlines have provided estimates of billing statement processing costs that range from $3.00 to $7.50 per statement. Be sure to consider this when setting up your billing practices.

Current Procedural Terminology (CPT) Codes

Just as the DSM-III-R provides us with diagnostic code numbers, there are code numbers designating the type of treatment given to a client. An early coding system, the RVS (relative value scale) assigned each treatment a five-digit code. On your insurance billing, instead of writing out the treatment, such as "50-minute psychological consultation," you would write "RVS 90803." Insurance companies provided RVS booklets to clinicians. The booklets included the RVS code, a description of the procedure, and specified how much the insurance company was willing to pay for the service. For example: "RVS 90803, one 50-minute-hour psychological consultation: 1.4." The 1.4 represented a unit of payment. In this way, insurance companies informed clinicians up front how much money they would pay for each unit. In this example, if a unit was equal to $50, the practitioner would multiply the RVS code unit of payment (1.4) times $50, which equals $70. After a long history of legal battles, eventually RVS codes and this unit pricing method were looked upon as medical price-fixing. In its place, we now have CPT codes.

CPT stands for physicians' Current Procedural Terminology. You may write or call the American Medical Association (P.O. Box 10950, Chicago, IL 60610; 800-621-8335) to request a copy of all CPT codes. When ordering a CPT manual, be sure to request the Evaluation and Management Services special supplement. This supplement gives the codes for administrative costs and procedures that some insurance companies will cover, such as photocopying records.

As with the RVS, the CPT consists of a five-digit number followed by an explanation of the treatment or procedure the code number reflects. It does not, however, include a unit of payment reflecting how much would be paid for that service. For example: "CPT 90841, Individual medical psychotherapy by a physician, with continuing medical diagnostic evaluation, and drug management when indicated, including insight-oriented, behavior-modifying, or supportive psychotherapy; time unspecified."

Keep in mind, if you are a nonmedical practitioner, that the CPT codes seem limiting because they reflect only the medical model.

Keeping Track of Income and Ongoing Expenditures

As an aid to knowing at a glance what your income is at any given time, you could keep a billing record book. This is used to keep a running tab of how much you have earned to date, without having to add up individual billing charts. The billing record is a three-column system. The first column is the amount charged, the second column is the amount paid, and the third column is the balance owed (see page 31).

To keep track of billing to insurance companies, I draw a line in the margin next to the billing date. This makes it easier to keep track of those clients with insurance and how often they are billed.

I also keep an accounts payable ledger in a columnar book for all of my expenses throughout the tax year. The columns from left to right include the following information:

Column 1:	Date
Column 2:	Payment Made To
Column 3:	Method of Payment (check number, cash, money order)
Column 4:	Amount Paid
Column 5:	Balance Due
Column 6:	Rent
Column 7:	Phones
Column 8:	Office Supplies
Column 9:	Office Decor/Furniture
Column 10:	Clerical
Column 11:	Testing
Column 12:	Consultations

			BILLING RECORD				Page:					

Client's Name:						Referred by:		
Spouse's Name:						Date of Referral:		
Address:						Billing Diagnosis:		
Client's ID No.						Year:		

Date of Service		Client(s)	Amt. Billed	Amt. Paid	Balance Due

Column 13:	Didactic Therapy
Column 14:	Entertainment
Column 15:	Transportation and Mileage
Column 16:	Practice Promotion
Column 17:	Cleaning and Maintenance
Column 18:	Public Liability Insurance
Column 19:	Professional Liability Insurance
Column 20:	Health Insurance
Column 21:	Retirement Plan
Column 22:	Seminars and Conferences
Column 23:	Literary Materials
Column 24:	Miscellaneous
Columns 25–27:	Comments or Explanations Regarding Expenses

I will not go into great detail about what is included in each of these columns. But, for example, Column 8, Office Supplies, includes stationery, stamps, billing envelopes, light bulbs, refreshments (e.g., coffee, tea, bottled water), tissues, note pads, and pencils.

Using this basic 27-column outline, you and your accountant should determine what to include in each column. (See Chapter 8, under "Accountants and Attorneys" for more discussion.) Although federal tax laws are the same for everyone, state tax laws and allowable expenses may differ. Also, the method of record keeping may differ from year to year. A consultation with your accountant at the beginning of each tax year will save you hundreds, if not thousands, of dollars and many hours by teaching you the proper notations for your expenses before the required year-end tax forms. A few hundred dollars spent with a reputable certified public accountant will make your practice inestimably more lucrative.

Of late there has been an increase in the number of simple, "user-friendly" software packages that practitioners can use for billing and maintaining accounting records. Programs such as Timeslips™ and Quickbooks™ from Intuit can help the practitioner who is not terrified of computers and enjoys handling his or her own finances. Others may find their accountants or bookkeepers already using this software.

How Not to Be Desperate

In an economy presently headed in a direction where people will have less, providers offering services that are not urgent may suffer a decrease in income. It takes faith in yourself and your abilities, as well as support from your friends, family, and fellow clinicians, to hang in there during your starting years and in times of economic slumps. Above all, it requires a sense of humor.

Keep in mind that being in private practice is entrepreneurial. Cash flow will vary, the number of billable client-hours will vary, and you have no control over the state of the economy. You must be aware of this when you enter the world of the private practitioner.

For the first two-thirds of my career, I held "second jobs" that were my primary source of income. For a number of years I saw a limited number of clients, keeping my practice to a few select hours two days a week. One of the best pieces of advice I can offer you is to start out using private practice as a secondary source of income. By not having to count on the income, you will not be afraid of losing a client.

Helmut Kaiser, a brilliant psychotherapist who died far too early, once said, in essence, that life is a constant battle between holding on to the secure and reaching out with risk, exploring our own curiosity. Kaiser called this a balance-in-tension between the known and the unknown. Keeping this balance-in-tension as a private practitioner is being able to go with the flow and bear the risk.

Critics will sometimes remark of a bad actor, "He shouldn't give up his day job." This might also apply to clinicians. If you need the security of a salaried income, take it—but balance it with reaching out with risk toward the unknown. I have found that all-or-nothing people generally end up with nothing. We must admit to ourselves that a person who spent years in college doing undergraduate and graduate work, who performed thousands of hours of internship with minimal or no pay, and who was willing to give up creature comforts for school and state examinations, gave up a lot in so thoroughly preparing for a world that can change overnight. Honor both the need for security and the need to reach out with risk.

3

Selecting Your Location

This chapter includes the importance of client accessibility to your practice, tips on selecting the proper neighborhood, and thoughts on maintaining client and therapist safety. The possibility of having more than one office and the pros and cons of practicing out of one's home are also discussed, along with the advantages and disadvantages of having your own, sharing, or subletting an office. What are the typical costs you can anticipate, and what are the hidden costs you may not have thought of? There will also be a discussion of my "by the hour" theory.

There are many important details to consider when choosing and moving into an office. Whether you choose to become the master tenant and lease space to colleagues, or to sublet an office in an already-existing practice, the following should be taken into consideration.

Business License

You need a city license, called a business and professional license, to start a business. In the Los Angeles area, this license generally costs between $35 and $40 a year plus one tenth of 1% of your total gross income. This figure will appear on your income tax; in Los Angeles the total fee cannot exceed $1,000 a year.

When considering different areas for locating your practice, first check with the city clerk to find out the cost of a business and professional license. This cost may be a significant factor in selecting a location.

The lowest fee for a business and professional license in Beverly Hills, for example, is $500.

Location

Clinician's ideas differ on this topic. In selecting a location for your practice, I suggest that you consider the following:

1. Determine the population center of the city in which you are going to practice. You can get this information by calling the chamber of commerce or a taxicab company. Situating your office according to population density means that travel time will be cut down for the majority of your clients. The population center of Los Angeles county, for example, is the corner of La Cienega and Wilshire boulevards. It is helpful to know where your office is located in relation to the densest population area of your city or region.

2. Some clinicians choose to practice in multiple settings, working certain days a week at one location and others at another location far enough away to attract a different client population. I recommend doing this, especially in the beginning of your practice. You will probably find that you attract more clients in one area than another, and can then decide whether you wish to concentrate on that area or continue splitting your time.

3. Accessibility to freeways is a consideration for most practices. However, if your caseload consists of many people who are not able to drive, you may want your office located close to public transportation.

4. Some clinicians believe you can charge clients more money if your office is in a prestigious neighborhood. Sometimes this is true. However, the cost of renting space, finding parking, and inadequate public access to your practice may offset the advantages of a prestigious neighborhood and, in the long run, make your overhead too high.

5. Whenever possible, find office space in a building that does not have other practitioners of the same type. This allows you to be unique in your setting and, as a result, may increase your referral base.

Many clinicians have offices in "shrink" buildings because the offices are designed specifically for them, with adequate waiting and consulting rooms. On the other hand, it can be advantageous to be the only psychotherapist on the block. I spend a great deal of time doing business with local vendors and often eat at neighborhood restaurants. The local merchants all know me by name, which makes me "the nearest game in town." Also, from a client's point of view, there may be negative stigma attached to a "shrink" building. Some people are very private and do not want to be seen entering a psychiatrists' building.

The reason "shrink" buildings exist is because many landlords do not want to rent to psychotherapists. They cannot get a percentage of your gross receipts, a condition often included in leasing agreements with retail business. The second reason is because they don't want "those nuts" coming in and out of their buildings.

If you present your practice as the outpatient clinic for every schizophrenic in town, you will be resented by other tenants in the building. This is one of the reasons why it is hard for therapists to rent office space in other than "shrink" buildings. When talking to your landlord or other tenants, be low-key about your business and respect your clients' privacy.

6. You may want to locate your office in a building with other healthcare delivery services so that you can maintain a steady flow of cross referrals. This consideration depends on the nature of the clients you intend to treat.

Distance is not always a disadvantage. I have a wealthy married client who drives an hour and a half to see me. Early in our session, I asked her why she drove so far to see a therapist and told her I could refer her to an excellent therapist closer to her home. She said the drive was her only opportunity to leave her home legitimately, and she spent the time organizing her thoughts. The long-distance drive also afforded her the excuse to go shopping in town and be on her own, away from her family. For this client, her therapy was a five- or six-hour process.

Crime Rate

Call the local police department of the area you are considering for your practice and ask for crime rates. Try to choose a low-crime area. Thieves tend to either target poor neighborhoods or go to places where they think there is a lot of money. Don't be fooled by a pretty building or a sales-happy realtor. Check with the local police department.

Pay attention to the outside of the building as much as the inside. Don't make the mistake of believing that because there is a great inside, the outside must be great as well. Visit your prospective office around the clock. This will allow you to test lighting and parking factors at night. Notice corner crevices where potential muggers can hide.

Although I do not recommend it, some therapists keep loaded guns in their offices. If it is common knowledge that you retain large amounts of cash given to you by your clients, you may be setting yourself up as a target.

The two break-ins at my office were made by thieves entering through a window. All my office equipment was stolen and drawers were emptied. Now, I live my life in consideration of the possibility that some-one may break in, and I have taken several steps to safeguard my office and the privacy of my clients' files. I requested an insurance broker to come to my office to assist in making the office more difficult for people to enter without my permission. I keep file drawers locked, and have recoded my clients' file names under a coding system used for insurance companies. I have also edited (using correction fluid) or removed in-criminating documents or letters given to me by clients, and I have in-stalled a wall safe to hold documents that cannot be altered. Many of my colleagues take controversial records home with them and place them in a locked file, but you may find this measure impracticable.

The Building

In selecting a building, safety is first and foremost. Pay attention to outside lighting, parking, and access routes to your office. Most clinicians select their office during daytime hours and then discover that the build-ing does not have the same services, accessibility, and feel during evening hours. Before deciding on an office, visit the building during day and evening hours, on weekdays and weekends, with the following in mind: Is there sufficient lighting inside and outside? Is there adequate street and public parking available? Are security and safety features sufficient, even outside normal business hours?

Consider what types of businesses you are located near and what types of businesses are in the neighborhood. If you were running an insurance agency and a primal-scream therapist had a practice next door, your nerves would probably be frayed by the end of the day. Try to situate your practice in an area of the building that allows for privacy.

If you need to maintain parking spaces, you will need a minimum of three: one for yourself, one for the client in session, and one for the arriving client.

Most therapists practice during both day and evening hours. As mentioned above, be certain your building maintains its services throughout. There are many horror stories about therapists who rented space in a building only to find it locked after seven o'clock at night, or that the air conditioning or heating was turned off during the hours when they saw the majority of their clients. One group of therapists had to pay $50 per hour to keep their office open and air conditioned after seven in the evening—and they discovered this only after they had signed the lease!

Accessibility and Parking

Parking problems are more severe than ever before. When I began my practice in the late sixties, the streets were accessible for parking and traffic was light. Nowadays, only permit parking is available on many streets.

Parking availability is very important, usually essential. Generally speaking, clients are insulted when they have to pay for parking. You may need to think creatively about such matters. Five popular restaurants are now located in the neighborhood of my office, which naturally makes parking a problem. I contemplated moving but decided first to approach one of the valet services. I arranged to have them park my clients' cars by offering a weekly payment to the valet service. I am now a therapist with valet parking.

The availability of parking is another good reason to visit your prospective office on the weekend. Circumstances could be totally different from the work week. For instance, if your office is in a residential area, the parking situation may be poor on the weekends because everyone is home and parking spaces are filled that are normally open during the work week.

Stairs and Elevators

If your practice includes or could include clients with physical injuries or disabilities, your office must be accessible via an elevator or ramp. If your clientele will not include people with physical limitations and your office has access by staircase only, check to see that your staircase is safe, clean, and well-lighted. Remember that people coming to see you are anxious. You can help reduce their anxiety by paying attention to this kind of detail.

Elevators can induce an enormous amount of anxiety in some people. In a sense, you are damned if you do and damned if you don't. Make sure the building has safety regulations posted in the elevator and that the elevator is in good working order.

A practice on the first floor eliminates the need for an elevator, but first-floor offices get more street noise and are easier targets for criminals.

Noise and Soundproofing

Therapists are often concerned that their sessions can be heard in either the waiting room or outside the offices, so they try to find a soundproof office. But offices are rarely truly soundproof. After 25 years of practice, I have yet to find a soundproof office.

One way to improve soundproofing is to install double-hung doors. Inexpensive to add, they create a vacuum between the doors that shuts out sound.

Another way to achieve the effect of soundproofing is through the use of strategic noise. Although you can purchase noise machines, one of the best ways to create strategic noise is with a radio. Place the speakers in the waiting room with the radio and controls in your office so that you can adjust sound levels. The radio noise ensures privacy for your clients in session. Never leave the volume or channel control in the waiting room. If you do, a waiting client who doesn't want to miss a ball game may decide to change the station, and this could be disruptive. Have your radio premarked and preset so that you can turn it on and know you have the same audio level.

Waiting room chairs are best placed facing the wall of the consultation room. This will seat those clients who are waiting at the farthest distance possible from the consultation room, where they will be less likely to overhear another's session. If clients in the waiting room hear something, they tend to projectively identify as if they were the client in session, and, thus, stop listening.

Do your best to protect a client's privacy by controlling noise in the waiting room by whatever method necessary. Conduct a trial run of your setup by having a few people talk or even yell in the consultation room while you remain in the waiting room. How much can you hear?

As important as controlling the sounds from within your office is controlling those sounds you will hear from outside your office during both day and evening hours. Spend different portions of the day and evening inside the office you intend to rent so you can listen for possible disruptions. An office with a great interior can become a nightmare if it's located on a main thoroughfare during peak traffic hours. Check it out in advance. The comfort that a quiet environment will grant both you and your clients is well worth the effort.

Climate Control

Two important things to look for in office space are being able to control the temperature and lighting. Look for an office that has both air conditioning and heating and has windows for cross ventilation.

It can be enormously uncomfortable to practice in an office without proper air circulation and temperature control. An office that is too hot, too cold, or stuffy is death to a private practice. Also, keep in mind that air-conditioning and heating systems can fail. Windows and a small electric heater are essential for such contingencies. Beware of modern sealed buildings in which you cannot open or close the windows.

Make sure you have access to the thermostat. If you cannot control the temperature after a certain hour because the thermostat is locked up, and you cannot open a window, you are in trouble.

Check that the air-conditioning system has a switch that allows you to block the air-conditioning vents between offices if necessary. Often air-conditioning vents are not evenly distributed throughout the office. Once you shut the outside door, it is 85 degrees on the inside and 60 degrees on the outside, or vice versa.

A good range for office temperature is 67 to 72 degrees. Keep blankets, sweaters, and a fan in the office for clients' comfort.

If you cannot control the temperature inside your office, then don't rent the office!

Light Control

The only thing you have to sell is service. Good service provided in an uncomfortable setting becomes bad service. When lighting is soft, it tends to open the iris in the eyes, and this creates more emotive responses. If you practice "feeling state" psychotherapies and you want to encourage catharsis, you could do so by darkening the room and having area lighting as opposed to bright overhead lighting. You must be able to control the lighting to be able to vary it from client to client.

Light has a great effect on people who are depressed. About 30% to 60% of the clients seen in private practice suffer from dysthymia and depression. This can be compounded by seasonal affective disorder, which typically lasts from November through April. One of the treatments for seasonal affective disorder is a light treatment in which the person spends an hour a day under special lamps.

The lighting in your office can also work to improve your abilities. Like many people, I suffer from biochemical depression. When the season changes, if I cannot control the light in my office, I tend to get depressed sometime between four and six o'clock in the afternoon. To work optimally, and to keep an effective balance in my life, I need to keep a constant amount of light in my environment.

Maintaining More Than One Office

At present, I have one office in Manhattan Beach and another in West Los Angeles. I financed the offices by putting up the capital for all the interior equipment (lights, office equipment, and furniture) and then leasing the offices on the days I was not using them. The majority of the costs of the Manhattan Beach office are picked up by my sublessee.

The pros and cons of leasing or subleasing include the following: As the lessor you are contractually obligated to a greater amount of money than as a sublessor. In addition, as a lessor, you may need to supply services (cleaning carpets, fixing broken locks) that your landlord may not wish to supply. Sublessors have less responsibility and will be more transient. In either case, whether you are a lessor or sublessor, establish in writing the degree of maintenance and service provided and expected.

You can also rent an office by the day. There are many offices available as sublets. Look in the advertisement sections of the publications of your state and local professional organizations.

Pros and Cons of Practicing Out of One's Home

Generally speaking, practicing from your home is not a smart idea. Therapists who practice out of their homes are leaving themselves open to trouble. Unless you have special facilities, there is no privacy for you, your family, or your clients.

I knew a professional couple who built a separate facility above their garage. This gave them an office that was disconnected from the house and where clients were able to enter and exit in privacy. A situation like this can work well, but is hard to find.

In the beginning of your practice, your clients will have different income levels and backgrounds and, as a beginning therapist, you may be less able to make early diagnoses. Be aware that you work in a dangerous business and that some people you treat can be dangerous: over 80% of homicides are committed by people who know one another! If people know where you live, they know where to find you. I advise you to not practice out of your home, particularly if you are just beginning your private practice. On rare occasions, I have seen an already-established client in my home, but never a new client.

Also be aware that, like your office practice, your home practice must be protected by public and professional liability insurance. The laws of your city may pose problems with respect to acquiring a business license for practicing your profession at home.

4

Setting Up Your Office

Once you have selected an office, it is time to think about the things you will need to practice in it. This chapter includes discussions of office layout, furniture, and telephone options such as answering machines, answering services, beepers, and the handling of phone emergencies and interruptions.

Timothy Leary, in his early work with the use of hallucinogenic drugs, stated that the hallucinogenic experience involved "set and setting" more than the ingestion of the hallucinogen. Likewise, when choosing a building or an office, you are choosing the environment for the "mind set" in which you provide services. An office or building that is disparate from the feeling tone you wish to create can greatly affect your practice.

Doors

Let's start with the first door the client enters. Along with your name, should your degree and specialty be displayed on the door? Unless you are counting on getting much walk-in traffic, I recommend having only your name on the door. Clients can feel self-conscious walking through a doorway labeled as belonging to a mental health professional. Again, be conscious of noise. A squeaky entrance door may be heard in the consultation room and can be a distraction from the session. Keep a can of metal lubricant in your office.

Next is the door between the waiting room and the consultation room. Remove all handles on the waiting room side of the door. There is nothing more annoying than a client who is new to your practice twisting and turning the knob on this door. Also place a "Please Do Not Disturb" sign on the door.

Finally, let's look at the exit or "escape" door. Some therapists believe that it is essential to have a door by which one client can leave without being seen by the next. Other therapists believe that escape doors add to the "shame factor" associated with seeing a psychotherapist. There are many points in favor of each position. You must also consider your clients' feelings when deciding whether to have an escape door.

I believe that constructing an escape door is essential to the maintenance of good psychotherapy for several reasons. First, many clients want the privacy. Second, clients may know one another through referral, and you may need to book their sessions back-to-back (though you should avoid this whenever possible). Third, many clients leave a session distraught and need the privacy afforded by an exit door. And finally, when I began my practice and didn't have an escape door, I found that I unconsciously attempted to have each session end "nicely." Later, though, I realized that ending a session on an up note may not be what the client needs at that time. Clients and therapists both need to realize that a therapy session is not a one-hour television show that always has a happy ending.

The illustration on the next page shows one arrangement for installing an escape door in a one-entrance office. Most landlords are willing to construct nonbearing walls with a door.

If the escape door opens into a hallway, always post a "Do Not Disturb" sign to discourage vendors and solicitors.

Furniture

The furniture in your office is related to temperature and comfort. On a hot day, leather furniture can be very uncomfortable. If possible, give your clients an option between leather or cloth furniture. Another important factor is to select furniture without buttons. Nervous clients have a tendency to pull buttons off furniture. If you include hypnosis or relaxation therapies in your practice, supportive, ergonomic furniture is important.

Although the choice of an office, its location, and its decor will probably not determine the type of therapy you practice, they can cer-

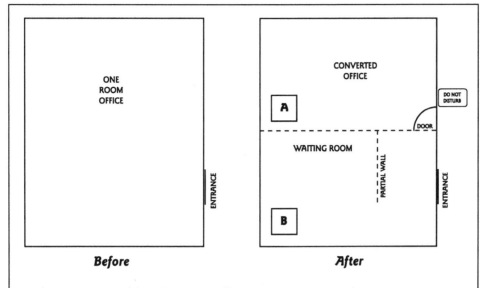

ONE
ROOM
OFFICE

CONVERTED
OFFICE

A

DO NOT
DISTURB

DOOR

WAITING ROOM

PARTIAL WALL

ENTRANCE

B

ENTRANCE

Before   ***After***

Add nonbearing walls to create an escape door.

Create an office and a waiting room. Client A can exit without being seen; client B has privacy in the waiting room.

Your landlord may pay for the installation of an escape door, especially if you have a long-term lease. If not, installing a nonbearing wall and door system can be amortized over a one-year period at less than $50 per month.

tainly have an influence. If you wish to practice psychodynamic psychology with a minimum of transference stimuli, a conservative approach towards your surroundings can assist your theoretical orientation. Likewise, an office that is reflective of your personality may encourage your client to make transferences based on your psyche rather than their own.

If you practice with a theoretical basis founded in counseling psychology (rather than clinical psychology), you may wish to have an office that focuses on comfort and encourages mutual exchange. A "den-like" setting might be appropriate for this theoretical orientation.

What is important to remember is that your office can tell your client a great deal about you. Pay attention to how your theoretical orientation is reflected in your professional surroundings.

If you are considering sharing an office, problems may arise concerning office decor. For instance, there are masculine-toned and feminine-toned offices. Likewise, if you and the clinician(s) you share with follow different disciplines, you will need to find an acceptable compromise. You may even find that you need to schedule extra transition time between clinicians to rearrange the furniture.

Shared Offices

If you share an office with another person and you both use it on the same day, time allocation may present another problem. Make sure you have a two-hour transition break. The first hour belongs to the earlier clinician, and the second hour belongs to the later. Reach an agreement at the outset to consider these hours as nonbookable. I also refer to this free-zone time as "pick-up hours," in which you can add an extra client into your day if needed. The clinician using the office in the earlier part of the day may need to schedule an emergency appointment or need an hour to complete paperwork. Likewise, the later clinician may need to schedule an extra hour at the beginning of the day, or may prefer to come in early to make calls and do paperwork. This two-hour leeway is necessary to prevent the confusion that can be created by trying to quickly change possession of the office, taking papers away, bringing papers in, and sorting out files.

Smoking Policies

As a healing-arts provider, you may specialize in helping people rid themselves of dangerous habits, such as drinking, smoking, and overeating. For those of you specializing in aversion therapy related to smoking, consider setting aside a room specifically for that purpose. With today's level of health consciousness, you will need to provide a smoke-free environment, and it may be appropriate for you to place a "no smoking" sign in your waiting room, especially if other clinicians share the room.

Smoking policies within the confines of your consultation room may vary. Formerly, in offices with proper ventilation, a client could choose to smoke or not, and any residual odor was sprayed with room deodorizer. Due to findings related to secondary smoke, you may want to ask clients not to smoke during sessions. If a client must have a cigarette during the course of a session, you can suggest taking a walk around the block.

The Telephone

People don't write when they want to see a therapist. For the foreseeable future, the telephone will continue to serve as the major link between the private practitioner and the client. Maintaining a phone number that remains with you throughout your practice is one of the most important investments you can make. If possible, have an answering machine attached to a phone other than your personal home phone so that you can separate business from personal calls. This also allows for easier accounting to the IRS at the end of the year.

As a teenager, I installed a telephone number in my parents' home. When I moved out of my family's home and rented my first college apartment, I took the phone number with me. I was able to do this because the area code remained the same. In the sixties, I transferred my phone number to an answering service in the area where the phone company would permit that number to continue. Up until the advent of call forwarding, I kept that same phone number as my answering service. With call forwarding, I was able to buy the number from the phone company and, for a service charge of less than $20 per month, it is now forwarded to my answering machine.

If you anticipate practicing within a 50-mile radius of where you began your practice, you can establish and own your own phone number. Having an answering service does not guarantee you your own phone number, especially if the answering service goes out of business. Having a constant phone number is an excellent business investment. If someone drops out of therapy for a while, then wants to return a year later, or misplaces your business card, only to find it while moving years later, the number will still be valid. Since I have been in practice for many years and have a constant number, I am now receiving phone calls from the children of clients I counseled 20 or 25 years ago. My current fee is $135 per 50-minute session, and the fee for maintaining my original phone number is under $20 a month, so it costs me less than two client-hours to maintain this service for one year. If I book two client-hours per year through the service, maintaining my original phone number has essentially paid for itself.

If you are a student, intern or trainee, or resident, and know in what city or area you are going to practice, I suggest you get your phone number now. Connect an answering machine to a phone in your home. If you already have this set up, then get a separate phone number and have this number answered by an answering machine or service. By maintaining a constant phone number, you become a psychological resource. Part of the business of private practice is being known as a psychological resource.

Whether you decide to get an answering machine, subscribe to an answering service, or hire a receptionist will depend on the nature of your clientele and your economic situation. Most nonmedical clinicians use either answering machines or answering services.

Local telephone companies now offer a variety of services that include receiving and sending messages, call forwarding, and even emergency contact. These services may be less costly than investing the capital in answering machines and beeper systems. Check with your local phone company to see what services they can provide, and compare the cost with that of answering machines, message services, pagers, and other equipment.

There are other factors to consider when choosing a service or answering machine. An answering machine enables you to listen to both the quality and content of what the client is saying. It also provides privacy, whether for famous people who do not wish to leave their name with an answering service or the nonfamous who demand that their therapy be kept in total confidentiality. You may choose to be available on an emergency basis via a beeper, but if you do not, having an answering machine allows you to choose when to return calls.

You may wish not to have your answering machine at your private practice because of possible interruptions during counseling sessions, especially if your office space is limited. Some clinicians prefer to have unlisted back-lines at their office so they can be contacted by already-established clients during the counseling day in case of last-minute cancellations or emergencies. If you decide on this method, ask that clients give your answering machine or service number for referrals, and check your answering machine for messages two or three times a day.

In light of some of the recent legislation being requested by representatives from federal agencies (such as the FBI and the CIA) about the potential accessibility of names, phone numbers, addresses, and the content of messages left on computerized message systems, you may wish to request a written statement regarding the confidentiality and accessibility of information that could be accumulated through use of these services.

The advantage of using an answering service is mainly its ability to contact you with complete messages through beeping services. Many people prefer using an answering service or receptionist because their clients speak with a live person.

Never share an answering service or machine with another clinician or any other person. It is an automatic breach of confidentiality if anyone else hears your clients' messages, except for the traditional exceptions of receptionists, secretaries, and administrative assistants.

Having visited many psychotherapists in the preparation of this book, I found that the single greatest breach of confidentiality in their offices are conversations between doctors and receptionists concerning clients' names, appointment times, and other information. I frequently heard, especially in psychiatrists' offices, receptionists shout messages such as, "Mr. Smith called," sometimes followed by very personal information.

If you need to talk with your secretary or receptionist, remember that it is illegal to disclose the names of anyone in your practice except under very special circumstances. Keep your voices low; others are listening and will projectively identify with the client being discussed, and become uncomfortable, to say the least.

A car phone, if you decide to have one, will enable you to check for messages and conduct business when stuck in traffic. Car phones in their current state are extremely expensive, since the owner pays for all incoming and outgoing calls. It is easy to run up a car phone bill to $600 to $700 a month, especially if you spend more than 20 minutes each way to and from work.

Emergency Numbers

Keep emergency phone numbers close to every phone. As well as the usual police, fire department, and other emergency services, it is a smart idea for mental health professionals to make a note of hotline and trauma center numbers that can serve as resources and consultation aids. Even during a typical therapeutic hour or when returning a phone call from a client, the necessity for these numbers may arise.

Phone Interruptions

The back-line in your office should have an on/off switch that can be turned off at the beginning and on at the conclusion of every session. In most practices, phone interruptions during sessions are unacceptable. Clinicians who complain of frequent emergency calls and phone interruptions must be encouraging them in some way. You get the calls you are willing to receive.

Files and Clinical Notations

Your clinical notations could someday be the deciding factor in a lawsuit against either you or your client. Casual "process notes" should be reviewed for potential implications by supervisors as well as interns. In some states, the law requires you to keep your notes for three years from

Page No.	CLINICAL NOTATIONS
Client's Name:	
Client's ID No.	
Year:	

• Client's remarks • Therapist's observations • Client's affect • Recommendations & interventions	
• Client's remarks • Therapist's observations • Client's affect • Recommendations & interventions	
• Client's remarks • Therapist's observations • Client's affect • Recommendations & interventions	
• Client's remarks • Therapist's observations • Client's affect • Recommendations & interventions	

the date of last service. Check with your local association to be certain of the requirements.

As a professional, you must view your records not only in the context of your client's present situation but also in view of years to come. This is especially true if these records are going to be left at a clinic without your direct supervision.

Remember, once you leave a clinical setting, all that is left of your work there is the recorded notation. Often, the therapist cannot be reached for a detailed explanation of what was written, and the notation must speak for itself.

For example, a student intern seeing a 16-year-old adolescent who discusses her fears about being a lesbian may make the notation "discussed lesbian tendencies in client." Years later, these notations may be reviewed by the government during a top-secret security clearance. Depending on the morality of the times, a security clearance may not be given due to such a notation.

A more appropriate clinical notation for the above example might be "client discussed feelings of sexuality and gender." This notation describes the kind and quality of the session without the possible condemnation of a homophobic investigating agent or agency.

In a private practice setting, therapists are in control of their files. The same does not hold true in a clinical setting. That's an enormous difference to keep in mind.

You can use a simple coding system for your client records. Here's a sample: 94-GOL-01. The first two numbers are the year of the beginning of treatment, the three letters are the first three letters of the client's last name, and the last two numbers are assigned in case there are two clients with the same three letters.

The Clinical Notations form is probably the most significant form you will fill out during the course of your practice, because this document can be admitted as evidence for and against your client in a court of law.

As a clinician, you may not have the right, based on the codes of evidence in your state, to withhold your notations or withhold giving a deposition. Tell your clients in advance that if they are going to be involved in any legal action (whether it be a car accident, a divorce, or buying the Brooklyn Bridge), they should inform you and give you permission in writing to speak to their representatives about matters of confidentiality as related to the field of psychotherapy within the laws of the state.

In every session I suggest that you follow the rule of thumb known as SOAP. Simply, this is:

S: notations about something the client SAYS
O: some aspect of the session the therapist OBSERVES
A: the client's AFFECT during the session
P: what you PRESCRIBE (your clinical suggestions)

The Clinical Notations form has a heading for client's remarks, therapist's observations, client's affect, and recommendations and interventions. The form is set up this way to remind you of the standard of practice. Check with your local association regarding standards of practice in your area.

The following should be listed on a clinical notation relating to an outside consultation: client's name and identification number; date; purpose of the consultation (medical, psychiatric, legal, testing, school, or other); consultant's name, profession, address, and telephone number; client's signature releasing confidentiality; and any comments.

5

Building Your Practice

This chapter includes discussion of business cards and the "scratch paper method" of using them; promoting your practice through newsletters and public speaking; and other methods of becoming visible. It also covers some referral services that are rarely considered.

Most mental health practitioners have spent many years in college and clinical training, cloistered from the world of marketing, merchandising, and entrepreneurialism. As a clinician in private practice, you will need to acquire these business skills to some degree, depending on how many other clinicians in your area are providing similar services and whether there are enough clients to go around. How much business skill you need will depend on local competition for services. Thinking of your practice in this way may be difficult, but it is essential for starting a successful business.

It takes about five years to build a private practice. One way in which you build your practice is by being visible. You are selling a service, and you need to market yourself and maximize what you have to offer. Ask an accomplished and knowledgeable professional for guidance and support, or contact a marketing consultant.

Specializations

If you want to build a private practice more quickly, specialize. Find a niche that no one else (or very few people) is filling and fill it. Specialization does not mean limiting yourself! You can be an expert to one group on one specialty and to another group on another specialty. For example, to some I am known as an expert on psychopathology; to others, I'm known as a consultant who works on television and theatrical projects. A career can have more than one focus.

If I were starting my career over, I might pursue the area of learning disabilities, which is still relatively untapped. I would probably open up a learning-disability center and hire teachers with expertise in attention deficit disorders, developmental disorders, and so forth. I would advertise through schools and local newspapers for specialists in the areas of reading and mathematics.

Another area to consider for specialization is workers' compensation. Some of the wealthiest therapists in Los Angeles are people who set up workers' compensation clinics and hire professional personnel. In other words, you can open a clinic and hire the experts you need; if you have the idea, someone else can supply the expertise. One example is a professional with a bachelor's degree in psychology who decided that the Hispanic workers' compensation market could be further developed; he now grosses approximately $1.7 million a year. Specialization can be very profitable.

You may start with several specialties until you find an area you love. Or you may find that your specialty is what makes you money, while work in another area excites you more but is not economically viable. My specialties happen to be what I love.

Target Your Market

You must target geographic areas where there is a market for psychotherapy. For example, in an area where there is a concentration of work in juvenile diversion, biofeedback, and hypnosis, you know there is a market for these services. You must also consider population density and whether there is room in that area for another therapist.

Be aware that certain cultures do not recognize psychotherapy as a legitimate, helpful tool. Also, some people will only visit a therapist of their own culture. If you speak a language other than English or have knowledge of a particular culture or ethnic group, advertise in publications that reach members of those populations.

Pros and Cons of EAPs and HMOs

Depending on your degree and license, you may be eligible to participate in Employee Assistance Programs (EAPs) and Health Maintenance Organizations (HMOs) within the service area of your practice. For a new clinician, these types of organizations can be a good way to establish a client base. For a more experienced clinician, it is a way to expand an existing client base. Contact local large businesses and talk to the people responsible for coordinating health services for the companys' employees.

EAPs and HMOs may require a yearly fee for you to advertise your name in their booklet of acceptable clinicians. There may be limits to the number of sessions a client can have or the amount of money you are allowed to charge.

Offering services to local HMO or EAP programs, such as conducting workshops on employer-employee relations or stress management, is an excellent way for you to get your name known, particularly if you have a specialty. Depending on your expectations of client referral, such promotional services are sometimes paid for and sometimes should be offered free of charge. Make sure clients referred to you and whose visits are paid for by these services can eventually belong legally and ethically to your private practice client base. Laws relating to this process differ from state to state.

Do not simply believe that what an EAP representative or brochure tells you is the law; check it out for yourself. Upon leaving a clinic, clinicians are frequently told they cannot take their caseload with them. Even though the clinic, EAP, or HMO may inform or contract you so that you are unable to take your caseload with you, such contracts or agreements may be illegal and unethical. In most cases, they are not binding. Consult your attorney before getting into a situation like this.

If you have just graduated or become licensed and are moving from a clinic setting or an EAP/HMO setting to a private practice, discontinuing treatment of your clients may not be in the clients' best interest. In some cases, it is unethical not to offer your clients the option of continuing treatment with you.

Becoming a Medicare Provider

Since July 1, 1990, psychologists and social workers have the option of becoming independent providers for Medicare. Although certain local requirements may differ from state to state and carrier to carrier, most will require that you request an application in writing.

The pros and cons of being a Medicare provider are no different from those of accepting payment from other third-party providers. You must decide whether you have the resources to fill out the appropriate paperwork and to stay updated on billing procedures and practices, and finally, if you wish to accept the reimbursement the provider has predetermined.

To apply for a Medicare provider number, start by calling the Social Security information number in your telephone book. You will be asked what city you practice in and given a number to call. When you call that number, you will reach the Part B Medicare Carrier. They will send you a Medicare provider number application, to be returned to the Certification and Profile Department.

In general, the request should include your name, address, specialty, tax identification number, and certification or license number. After you have sent this information, a formal application will be sent to you. Billing forms are available through the Government Printing Office in Washington, D.C. If you wish to order by credit card, call (202) 783-3328, and expect delivery in three to four weeks. If you wish to send a check, make it payable to the Superintendent of Documents and mail it to: U.S. Government Printing Office, Washington, DC 20402. Mail orders generally take four to six weeks.

With national health insurance looming on the horizon, everyone must stay informed about these issues. By reading association journals and attending association-sponsored and recommended workshops and conferences, we can make more informed decisions regarding the nature of our practice and the clientele we serve.

Using the Scratch Paper Method

Handing out your business card when introducing yourself to someone is a common procedure. The purpose of a business card is to inform people that you do psychotherapy. Your card should include your name, your highest degree, your address and phone number, and any legal designation required by the state.

To increase your visibility, use your business card as scratch paper. When writing someone a note or other information they have requested, use the back of your business card. The person taking the card will turn it over and notice that you work in the psychology field.

Don't hoard your business cards as if you are waiting for someone to approach you looking for a therapist. The purpose of a business card is to be sure your name is seen by as many people as possible. Using the scratch paper method, for example, I comfortably pass out over 1,000 cards each year.

If you are a psychology student, you should have calling cards that inform people that you are a student studying psychology. Your card should include a phone number that you maintain throughout your career (discussed in Chapter 4). From the beginning of your academic career, people should know that psychology is your field. However, you must make sure that your cards never misrepresent your academic level or license. Regulations regarding the advertising of psychological services are extremely strict (see Appendix A). Check with your state and local associations.

Remember, as a student of psychology, you already know more than the general public. Even though you cannot perform psychological services, you may be able to direct people to appropriate resources. As a result, you will start to be perceived as a psychological resource. Letting people know that you and psychology are related is the beginning of a career. The cost for business cards is minute compared to the cost of your education. Carry your calling cards with you at all times.

Increasing Your Exposure

Building a private practice is cumulative and geometric; it is not arithmetic. An arithmetic progression is one plus one plus one; a geometric progression is one times two times two. If each client tells two friends, who tell two friends, who tell two friends, your client base will soon be quite impressive.

Over the last 25 years, I have built a client base of approximately 14,000 people. This figure does not include students or referral sources. From day one I perceived myself not as a clinician looking for a client, but as a psychological information center and phone book. When speaking, I tell my audience to call me if they need help in any area. I let them know that I can be used as a resource directory. Now I am often asked if I am available for a consultation.

This information service helps people and builds your practice in two ways. First, people remember that you directed them to appropriate help. Second, the professional you have referred them to becomes aware of you and may reciprocate. Be aware that when you give someone your phone number, often two years will pass before they call you. That is what makes your permanent phone number so important.

Advertising

Without being in the phone book and without advertising, I believe it takes five years to fill 25 hours. If you want to build your practice more quickly, advertise your specialty—hypnosis, biofeedback, pain management, or whatever it may be. These specialties are areas of quick turnover, and new clients will find out you also do psychotherapy. What you are trying to do is to become visible.

Before planning an advertising campaign, check with your state and local associations about local advertising restrictions. Make sure you know what titles you may legally use, what services you may offer, whether your state license number must appear in advertisements, and, if you are an intern, whether you must list your supervisor's name in all advertisements.

If you choose to be in the public eye, whether through writing, lecturing, or appearing on local or network television as an expert, it is helpful to have an 8 by 10 portrait (color or black-and-white) for promotion and advertisement purposes.

Handouts

Whenever I have a speaking engagement, I always hand out a cartoon of a man standing on a soapbox holding a sign that reads: "The world is not coming to an end. Learn to cope!" People love to photocopy this and hand it out at work. Since my name and phone number are on the cartoon, they reach many people this way. Think of ways like this that you can reach a large audience; it may be as a lecturer, a columnist in the local paper, or a performer. Know yourself and your vulnerabilities: develop your own style. As long as your name and number reach people, this approach helps build your private practice. When speaking in front of a group, remember that you are not looking for clients, you are there to inform people about a subject in which you have expertise. Either attach your card to or type your name and number on a handout or something else that people can take away with them.

Once established, you can consider opening your own publishing company for printing materials you use at your seminars. A handout can be published rather inexpensively. The miracle of desktop publishing is a big plus in starting up, maintaining, and increasing your practice.

By using a handout when lecturing, I do not have to hand business cards at the end of the talk. Also, potential clients who might not otherwise approach me in a public setting will be able to get in touch with me. Some examples of handouts I use can be found in Appendix C.

Newsletters

If you are not computer literate, find a friend, associate, or colleague in a related field who will aid you in producing a newsletter. When using a personal computer and a speedy print shop, the production and mailing of a monthly newsletter can be inexpensive.

Newsletters can include articles, suggestions, ideas, reviews of books, and other therapeutic services that publicize your name to both past and present clientele, as well as to colleagues, local schools, churches, and any other organization that may post a one- or two-page newsletter.

You can further disseminate information about your practice by asking other clinicians or professionals to contribute articles to your newsletter. An attorney or accountant may provide you with helpful hints and tax tips relating to your clients' financial situations.

Other Referral Sources

Ten years ago, the city of Chicago instituted a program to teach bartenders how to recognize substance abusers and how to counsel people. Bartenders were paid extra money for having this knowledge. They felt proud to be a part of this program of intercepting alcoholism. Programs such as this are excellent, specific sources for referrals.

Manicurists, hairdressers, physical trainers, and other service providers are also referral resources that can be easily overlooked. People in these professions often have privileged access to private information and are in a position to refer their clientele to you. It pays to have lunch with people in service-related industries. Other sources of referrals include local institutions (schools, churches, hospitals) and allied professionals (people in the legal, medical, and social work fields).

Please do not limit yourself to the referral sources listed here. They have worked for me, but there are many more that could be at least as effective for you. As an example, I am currently supervising a clinical intern with a vast background in pediatric encorprisis and enuresis. He has decided to do a direct mailing to every pediatrician in the county explaining how he may be of service to them in a problematic area that supports their practice. Your own particular background can be your richest source of referral ideas. If you have experience in a particular profession, think of ways it can be related to the delivery of psychological services.

And remember, referring to other clinicians brings referrals back to you.

6

Making Your Practice What You Want It to Be

This chapter covers techniques on how to handle your thriving practice once you have built it. It includes a discussion of the screening process, deciding what kind of clients you want, and establishing your fees. Also discussed are that crucial first contact, and some additional thoughts on the therapist's responsibility to clients, as well as the client's responsibility to the therapist.

The Screening Process

Do not screen prospective clients over the phone. Not only is it difficult to get a fair idea of someone over the phone, it is considered solicitation of business and is against the law. A client must make the first contact. The only exception is an emergency involving guardianship issues (a parent calls about a 13-year-old child, for example, or someone calls regarding an elderly parent), and even then it is the guardian, not you, who should make the first contact.

Occasionally, a prospective client will try to engage you in a long conversation over the phone. Remember that your services are for sale, and follow these two policies: never talk on the phone longer than three minutes, and always follow the preceding policy.

If you get a referral call, accept the call and schedule an appointment with the person. As part of your initial phone contact, ask the prospective client to bring along any information necessary for filling out insurance forms. In addition, ask the person to write out and bring a list of any current medications, medical problems, and names of clinicians he or she is currently seeing.

Inform new clients of your exact session time (for example, explain that you see clients at 10 minutes past the hour as opposed to on the hour). For first appointments, ask prospective clients to arrive early to allow time to fill out paperwork prior to the first consultation.

The Dos and Don'ts of the First Contact

It is a good policy never to return a phone call from a new client until 24 hours after the first contact. This tells the prospective client that you are busy, and not desperate for clients. However, do return the call the next day, within 24 hours of the initial contact. Remember, this policy relates to new clients. Until the four-session trial period (discussed in the next chapter) is over, I recommend that you remain inaccessible unless very special circumstances occur. Some clinicians accept every call; that is their prerogative and another style of operating. I feel, though, that this policy can too easily get out of hand; you may soon find that you talk to your client more on the phone than in the office.

If necessary, current, long-standing clients can have your back-line office number and, if you choose, your private home number, so that they have 24-hour access. Clients should be encouraged to use those numbers at their discretion, before a situation escalates. If your definition of an emergency is a life-or-death situation, make this known to your clients. Medical physicians also find this approach effective.

If you choose to be available on a 24-hour emergency basis, use an answering service, one of the new services provided by various telephone companies, and/or carry a beeper. This way you will receive a detailed message on your client's current status and whereabouts. Also, if an emergency arises, the lag time between your client's call and the beeper transmission acknowledgment will be less than one minute. Any other procedure is insufficient.

If you want to find out about the best answering services and beepers available from first-hand experience, talk to a medical internist or a prominent cardiologist in your area.

What Kind of Clients Do You Want?

It is important to establish a client base with the greatest potential for future referral of clients you want to treat, according to your specialty, your clinical skills, and your ability to treat specific disorders.

For example, I want to focus on counseling psychology issues, treating people whose dysfunctions or disorders fall within the scope of a general counseling practice. I do not wish to be a clinician who is available on a 24-hour-a-day basis treating seriously distraught and disabled clients. So, I have chosen not to see nonmedicated psychotics or any practicing substance abuser unless he or she is willing to enter a treatment or networking program within 30 days of our first session.

When thinking of accepting referrals and referral resources, ask yourself the following questions. Do you want:

- to treat only people in certain professions?

- to focus on a specific ethnic or religious group?

- to focus on one gender?

- to treat only insurance-based clients?

- to target a particular economic strata of clientele?

- to specialize in the treatment of a specific disorder? If so, do you want to treat only the person with the disorder, or also the people affected by the person's disorder?

Treating your desired clientele may limit your client caseload at first. However, it may also permit you to live the life you want and need to live. Your needs are one of the most important factors to consider while building your private practice. It can determine whether you run your practice or your practice runs you.

Establishing Fees

One of the first questions asked by new interns is "How much should I charge?" One method is to find out the average fee charged by similar professionals working within a 50-mile radius of your location. You can get statistics from articles or by calling the research department of your state association. I generally recommend to interns (prelicensures) that they charge somewhere between 50% and 75% of the typical and usual fees for services from a fully licensed practitioner.

Today, in most metropolitan areas, the average fee charged by non-medical, licensed mental health professionals is around $75 to $100 per 50-minute session. At the start of a private practice, I advise interns to charge between $50 and $75 per session. Many interns respond to this advice by exclaiming, "But I'm getting most of my clients from the clinic where I worked, and I've only been receiving 5, 10, or 15 dollars a session. My clients can't afford that!" But as I stated in Chapter 1, you must charge what you wish to earn, not what you think you are worth. One of the most important techniques in the business and economics of delivering a professional service is establishing a fee. Once that fee is established, you may—because you are trying to build a practice or because you would like to work with a particular person—negotiate and accept any fee that meets your needs in that situation. But first establish your fee in your mind as well as in your clients' minds.

You will see that the economic structure of your practice begins to change as your clients refer people who can pay your established fee. Let your clients know that private practitioners usually cost significantly more than what is charged by public clinics or hospitals for outpatient services. They will appreciate that you are giving them a discounted rate.

In the beginning of a psychotherapeutic relationship, it is a clinician's responsibility to set clear boundaries relating to time, money, and procedures for client/therapist contact. At the same time, our clients need to be responsible to us. We are essentially being hired as independent contractors to provide professional services. As the employer, the client is responsible for adequately and promptly compensating the therapist for services rendered.

Discuss your fee openly, and make it clear that you expect the client to uphold his or her side of the arrangement. You do not need a complex sliding-fee scale, but it is a good idea to take the client's economic circumstances into account. You may also wish to allow clients a pro bono first session. Some clinicians disagree with this position, feeling that a clinician should be paid for every hour of client contact. While this is true and certainly encourages client responsibility from the outset, your private practice is a business, and the consumer has a right to initial access without a fee.

Changing Fees

Whether you are changing your fees due to the economic pressures of rent, general cost-of-living increases, or whether you simply wish to earn more money, I recommend that you check first with your state association regarding your legal and ethical responsibility to a client who will not be able to meet your anticipated fee hike. Then decide whether you are willing to keep your entire clientele at your current rate even if some can afford the fee increase. If you decide to raise your fees, consider how best to handle those clients who cannot afford the increase. Whenever possible, give your clients plenty of advance notice (at least 60 days), and have available the names of at least three clinicians or agencies that can provide psychotherapeutic services at your old fee or lower. Finally, make it known that when your clients refer a new client to you, they should either have the new person speak to you about fees or state your new established rate.

Sometimes, unexpected circumstances will force you to change your fees. In 1986, my office building changed owners, and I was given 90 days to negotiate a lease at the new, higher rate or leave. I priced available, comparable office space and decided that what the new landlord was requesting was on the high side but reasonable.

By dividing my new rent by the number of clients I was seeing, I found that if my clients could pay $5 to $10 more per session, I would essentially be earning the same income, staying in my old, familiar offices. I discussed this change with my clients and asked them to let me know within 30 days whether or not they could afford an additional $5 to $10 charge. Within two weeks most of my clients informed me that they could afford this fee increase. Some, however, could not. Ultimately I decided to continue charging sessions at the old rate and build an annual cost-of-living increase into my fee, rounding the figure to the nearest multiple of five. My clients agreed, and to this day, I maintain the same offices.

I have known many psychotherapists who have bartered their services. However, in 1992 the State of California Board of Behavioral Science Examiners revoked a psychotherapist's license, finding that bartering or exchanging services represents a dual relationship. In this particular case, the psychotherapist was exchanging therapeutic services for weekly housekeeping services. Check with your state and national associations, as well as your licensing boards, to see to what extent bartering is or is not be acceptable.

The Introductory Packet

The State of California Board of Behavioral Science Examiners suggests that clinicians place a resume or curriculum vitae in a client's introductory packet to ensure that the public knows the clinician's academic and clinical background. In addition, certifications and licenses should appear on waiting room or consultation walls. Before a first session, you can leave an introductory packet in the waiting room for a prospective client.

Some suggestions for what to include in this packet are your curriculum vitae, the Client's Bill of Rights, the Confidential Patient Information form. After interviewing the client, you may decide to include additional forms such as the Consent for Release of Confidential Information, the Limits of Confidentiality, and the Authorization to Obtain Confidential Information. (All these forms are discussed below.)

Place the forms in a folder and, if you do not have a receptionist who can hand the folder to the patient, attach the folder to a clipboard with a pencil and leave it in the waiting room. Attach a brief note to the folder asking the client to please fill out and sign the forms. Never write the client's name on this note; use only the person's initials. Before the appointment, write the amount you usually charge and the time limits of your consultation in the folder.

Curriculum Vitae

Several years ago there was talk among the legislature about requiring professionals to give a curriculum vitae to all new clients and patients. To my knowledge, this discussion got lost in the shuffle.

Since the beginning of my practice, I have included a copy of my CV and biography in my introductory packet. Those of you who practice using analytic orthodoxy may not wish to do so, but I believe that all practitioners should have their CV or abbreviated biography available for their clients.

The biography can also be used as an insert in workshop booklets and in handouts given to attendees of your lectures and speaking engagements. (See Appendix D for examples of curriculum vitae formats.)

Client's Bill of Rights

The Client's Bill of Rights discusses consumer protection and what therapists are not allowed to do. Some states require or will be requiring the clinician to post or hand out booklets, or have prospective clients sign forms, on ethical and unethical practices. Clinicians will also be required to inform the client where breaches of ethics can be reported. Your state and local associations or your state licensing board can give you this information.

Consent for Release of Confidential Information Form

The Consent for Release of Confidential Information form is used for consultations with other professionals or with persons other than your client. It addresses information that cannot be held confidential under state law.

This form can also be used in couples and family counseling. Simply ask all parties involved in conjoint and family sessions to sign this release. It must be clear to them that you cannot maintain confidentiality or privilege due to the possibility of triangulation, which can occur when doing therapy with more than one client at a time. For example, you can be triangulated by a simple two-minute phone call when one client calls to "secretly share some personal information." This can potentially be perceived by other clients as withholding and, therefore, a betrayal of their trust.

I once read that "Good judgment comes from experience and experience comes from bad judgment." I strongly recommend that the Consent of Release of Confidential Information form be signed by clients in conjoint family therapy.

Limits of Confidentiality

The Limits of Confidentiality form is not required by law, but I believe a client should give informed consent before a consultation. I believe it is ethical to inform a prospective client that there are limits to confidentiality, so I will not talk to any prospective client until this form is signed. The opposing view is that signing this form will lead a client to withhold important information that must be reported for the health and safety of others, such as child abuse and elder abuse.

Client's Bill of Rights

You, the client, have the right to:

- receive respectful treatment that will be helpful to you

- receive a particular type of treatment or end treatment without obligation or harassment

- a safe environment, free from sexual, physical, and emotional abuse

- report unethical and illegal behavior by a therapist

- ask questions about your therapy

- request and receive full information about the therapist's professional capabilities, including licensure, education, training, experience, professional association membership, specialization, and limitations

- have written information about fees, methods of payment, insurance reimbursement, number of sessions, substitutions (in cases of vacation and emergencies), and cancellation policies *before* beginning therapy

- refuse electronic recording, but you may request it if you wish

- refuse to answer any questions or disclose any information you choose not to reveal

- know the limits of confidentiality and the circumstances in which a therapist is legally required to disclose information to others

- know if there are supervisors, consultants, students, or others with whom your therapist will discuss your case

- request, and in most cases receive, a summary of your file, including the diagnosis, your progress, and type of treatment

- request the transfer of a copy of your file to any therapist or agency you choose

- receive a second opinion at any time about your therapy or therapist's methods

- request that the therapist inform you of your progress

© 1989, California Association of Marriage and Family Therapists. Reprinted from The California Therapist, *the publication of CAMFT, Nov/Dec 1989, by permission.*

CONSENT FOR RELEASE OF CONFIDENTIAL INFORMATION

I,_____ hereby authorize and request that
(Client's Name)

_____

(Clinician's Name)

may release all confidential professional information pertaining to me (or my minor children) to

_____

_____

_____

I understand that I may revoke this consent at any time by informing the above parties

in writing.

In consideration of this consent, I hereby release the above parties from any legal

liability for the release of this information.

Signature _____   Date _____
(Client)

and/or

Signature _____   Date _____
(Parent or Guardian)

Limits of Confidentiality

Information discussed in the therapy setting is held confidential and will not be shared without written permission except under the following conditions:

1. The client threatens suicide.

2. The client threatens harm to another person(s), including murder, assault, or other physical harm.

3. The client is a minor (under 18) and reports suspected child abuse, including but not limited to, physical beatings, and sexual abuse.

4. The client reports abuse of the elderly.

5. The client reports sexual exploitation by a therapist.

State law mandates that mental health professionals may need to report these situations to the appropriate persons and/or agencies.

Communications between the clinician and client will otherwise be deemed confidential as stated under the laws of this state.

Having read and understood the above, I agree to these limits of confidentiality.

_____   _____
Name of Client or Guardian   Date

_____
Signature of Client or Guardian

_____
Signature of Clinician

Authorization to Obtain Confidential Information

The Authorization to Obtain Confidential Information form is to be used for clinical notes on clients, for example when you contact a client's doctor and inform him or her that the client has come to you for psychotherapy. You can then ask the client's doctor pertinent questions relating to the case. Be sure to record all names of persons you speak with in relation to your client.

I understand and appreciate those clinicians working within the psychoanalytic mode who choose to limit the amount of information they give to their prospective clients so as not to interfere with transference processes. Nevertheless, whether that information is about the therapist or about the limitations of psychotherapy, an informed client is better able to consume psychotherapeutic services than an uninformed client.

With the increase in mandatory reporting of certain acts committed by or against clients, the concept of a truly confidential client/therapist relationship no longer exists. It is my opinion that the state and many professional organizations have wrongly insisted upon the reporting of incidents. Reporting discourages clients from seeking help, and in many instances only further damages the people that the reporting laws are intended to protect.

I believe the civil right of privacy outweighs society's need to know, and that the trend in our profession is toward hysteria. This hysteria is based on the naive belief that the reporting of information to police or governmental agencies has a positive effect on most clients. I am fully aware that there are situations in which children, spouses, and the elderly must be removed from environments that are dangerous to their well-being. I also understand that not reporting could result in greater damage or even the death of a client or someone in the client's life. The decision about whether or not other institutions or individuals should be informed should be left to the discretion of the clinician, with or without the client's permission.

It is my conviction that as professionals we must choose what we believe is politically and morally correct and practice accordingly. I hold the right to privacy above these other considerations and believe that the so-called ethical thrust toward reporting is yet another attempt by the state to violate citizens' civil rights.

AUTHORIZATION TO OBTAIN CONFIDENTIAL INFORMATION

I, _____ , hereby authorize and request that
(Client's Name)

_____
(Name of Information Source)

_____
(Address and Phone Number)

may release all confidential medical, psychological, psychiatric, educational, and/or other
appropriate information acquired in the course of my evaluations and treatments (or those of
my minor children) to

_____
(Clinician's Name)

I understand that I may revoke this consent at any time by informing the above parties
in writing.

In consideration of this consent, I hereby release the above parties from any legal liability for
the release of this information.

Signature _____   Date _____
(Client)

and/or

Signature _____   Date _____
(Parent or Guardian)

Phone Sessions

I prefer face-to-face clinical contact with my clients. Yet, at times, I hold full 50-minute sessions over the telephone. There are some clinicians whose entire practice is phone-based. Depending on your clientele, their diagnoses, and your treatment style, phone sessions are a matter of professional preference and ethical consideration. Quality therapy can be delivered in person or by telephone.

The pros and cons of phone therapy relate to the boundaries a therapist needs to establish. I have found that the degree to which a prospective client insists on taking a lot of time during the initial phone contact reflects the amount of control the client will assert, as well as the client's potential to attempt to stretch the boundaries of psychotherapy.

Phone therapy with already-established clients can be very effective. I see many clients whose work does not permit them as many in-office sessions as their need for clinical contact warrants. I have found that by combining phone contacts with in-office contacts, their success ratio is similar to those whose therapy is limited to in-office contact. Also, remaining in touch for five minutes a day with a client who is going through an extremely difficult period (such as surgery, medical testing, or divorce) reduces the stress of the event and establishes a strong and positive transference.

Clinicians should remain aware that frequent phone calls from a client may mean that the in-office psychotherapy is not an effective treatment for the client's disorder. Helping clients develop a social/psychological network may be extremely important, especially if you are working with substance abusers who are new to recovery.

7

Managing Your Time

This chapter discusses several techniques and considerations in scheduling your clinical day. These include the length of sessions, how to prevent overload, seasonal considerations, the client- hour, and other time-related topics.

Putting Things in Perspective

Time is a pressing consideration in all of our lives. It is probably the only commodity we cannot really save. The issue of time in therapeutic sessions has been discussed in thousands of books and articles. In this section, I address the issues that I have found to be the most important elements of the time factor in running a private practice.

A focused relationship, in which people are genuinely engaged in listening and responding, leaves us with the experience of being known, as if we have spent a lot of time with that person. Quality time is focused, engaged, and attentive.

Psychotherapy has shown me the power of quality time. For example, after seeing a client for three months in one 50-minute session per week, I demonstrate the importance of this focused, engaged, and revealing interaction by sharing the fact that we have only been in one another's presence for a total of 12 hours. Using our relationship as a reference allows me to introduce the concept of quality, or focused, time. At this time I can focus on the impact of an "engaged encounter."

Scheduling Clients

In the beginning of your private practice and throughout an already-developing practice, you will find yourself booking several first-time clients within the same time period. Since there seems to be a rhythm or series of phases to the psychotherapeutic process, I would like to provide a word of caution. If the majority of these first timers decide to stay with you in an extended psychotherapeutic relationship, you may find yourself alternately elated and burnt out by having a group of clients that is going through the same phase of therapy at the same time.

We are all aware of the therapeutic honeymoon. In the early phase of psychotherapy, when positive transference is established, sessions will tend to proceed with a great deal of ease. Within 60 to 90 days, the honeymoon will wane, and clients may begin to report the following sentiments:

- I've taken 3 steps forward and 12 steps back.
- At first I thought our seeing one another would help, but it obviously hasn't.
- You promised . . .
- I expected . . .

If you maintain a caseload of 15 to 25 client-hours per week, having five or six clients presenting this early phase of therapy at the same time can cause you a great deal of stress. In the first 60 to 90 days, you may feel elated by receiving a substantial increase in clientele and encountering the ease of the early sessions. Although you may not be able to control how many new clients you accept at a single time, especially early in your practice, please be aware that you can be setting yourself up for a situation in which you find yourself being placed on a pedestal with early positive transference from several clients and then three months later being "devalued" by the same group. Awareness of this situation can moderate your feelings of elation at having a new group of clients, as well as moderate your countertransference at being devalued. With the exception of those who can control client flow, this phenomenon seems to affect all clinicians. Being aware of this clinical phenomenon is your best defense, especially if you are maintaining one hour per week with a didactic, supervising psychotherapist.

Rudolph Eckstein, one of our premier child psychoanalysts, stated in a series of lectures that therapists don't do a lot of work for the first two years of therapy. After this time, the client stops bringing in daily events and will turn to "the issues." This, Dr. Eckstein says, is when the therapist must really go to work.

Four-Session Evaluation

One policy that can help in dealing with the rhythms of psychotherapy is to have four consultations with a new client and then to decide, with your client, whether or not to continue the relationship. At times a four-session evaluation is not sufficient, but usually you will know by then whether or not you can help the person. At this point, the client also has a sense of how well you work together.

Interaction between yourself and a prospective client should indicate to you whether or not you can treat the person. This assessment will sometimes happen after the first session, sometimes in later sessions. I advise clients during our first session that we should explore their problems and possible solutions, and, at the end of the third or fourth session, decide whether or not I am the appropriate clinician to meet their needs.

The 60-Minute Hour and Other Myths

The idea that a session should begin on the hour is one of the worst ideas ever to hit our field. This concept conforms to industrial-age thinking and has little to do with the human psyche or urban reality. The length of a session is a matter of tradition and acculturation. In the United States right now, the typical length of a psychotherapy session is 50 minutes.

If you run a 50-minute session, begin your session at 10 minutes after the hour. This serves several purposes. When you begin the session at 10 minutes after the hour, your clients will perceive of their appointments, beginning on the hour (e.g., a 5:10 appointment is thought of as a 5 o'clock appointment) and, as a result, few clients will ever be late for a session. Also, a client's travel time to your office may be affected as much by traffic conditions as by distance. These conditions are not within the control of your client. Thus, you will be able to differentiate between passive-aggressive clients who "keep you waiting" and clients who genuinely have difficulty reaching your office on time.

By starting a session 10 minutes after the hour, you will end your session on the hour. Since most clients will "hear" a 5:10 appointment as a 5:00 appointment, they will tend to arrive on time. As a result of schooling, television, and other social structures, most clients find ending a session on the hour natural. Scheduling sessions this way reduces the time problems that starting on the hour and ending ten minutes before the hour can create.

Most clients actually need longer than the 50 minutes designated as a client-hour. These "hours" are referred to as "sessions." If you refer to your session as an hour, your clientele will literally expect a 60-minute session. Watch your use of these terms. If you see clients for less than 60 minutes, get out of the habit of referring to your session as an hour. This terminology can be misleading, particularly when quoting fees over the telephone. Tell prospective clients that you charge, for example, $75 for a 50-minute session. Make it clear exactly how long your sessions run.

Knowledge of your own limitations will help you to see as few or as many clients as you wish in a day. It will also help you to determine how many days a week to practice. Since one of the purposes of your practice is to provide you and your family with a comfortable lifestyle, time and money are serious issues.

Most appointments are booked according to the numbering structure of appointment books. A recent study showed that people with appointment books numbered from seven in the morning until seven at night worked longer days than people in similar occupations whose appointment books were numbered from eight in the morning until six at night. Whether this is some form of a projective test (to see how long you and I want to work), or whether it's a conspiracy by appointment book companies to have us work more hours so that we can pay for the ever-increasing costs of appointment books, I don't know.

Some people enjoy working longer hours and fewer days. If you do, it helps to book clients based on their diagnosis.

There is no doubt that some sessions should last for two or three hours and others should stop after five minutes. Be aware that the therapeutic process runs hot and cold for clients as well as therapists. One session may be uneventful, but the following session may bear amazing fruit.

Booking by Diagnoses and Biorhythms

Since most psychotherapy is conducted on a once-a-week basis, you will find that certain rhythms exist both in you and in your clientele. Use your knowledge of these rhythms when scheduling clients.

The number one way to prevent burnout is to book your sessions according to diagnosis. Especially if your caseload is large or if you have clients who tend to debilitate therapists (i.e., borderlines), you may want to book clients based on their diagnosis and in relation to your own energy level. For example, do not schedule several people with similar depressive syndromes one after another. Also, if you recognize certain times as your least therapeutically creative hours and yet, due to either economic or clinical necessity, must see clients during that period, select clients who will bring energy to the session. My daily rhythm is lowest between four and six o'clock in the afternoon, so I like to book talkative clients at that time. I do not see depressives after seven o'clock at night.

By regulating the lighting in your office and keeping it consistent, you can control one variable helpful in encouraging emotional states. Clients with certain diagnoses feel different during different times of the day. Some depressives tend to feel bad in the morning; as the day progresses, they feel better. With other depressives, the opposite may occur. During your intake and diagnostic interviews, find out whether your clients notice patterns to their feelings based on time of day. You and the client may be able to select a time of day when he or she will be more receptive to the psychotherapeutic process.

Staying On Time

Staying on time is very important. It is courteous to your client in the waiting room. It is also courteous to you, giving you 10 or 15 minutes to relax, use the restroom, make necessary calls, or do necessary paperwork.

A practice usually runs more smoothly and feels less rushed when you inform your client five minutes before the session ends that there are only a few minutes left. Time problems can occur with transference and countertransference issues when clients are obsessive/compulsive or have paranoid personality disorders. The issues that cut to the heart of these clients are always time and money.

Give yourself a break if every so often you find yourself running over. We are not machines. Our clients are not machines. An extra minute or two is sometimes necessary to help clarify or express an important idea in a session summation. However, when a client introduces a different or new topic for discussion within five minutes of the end of the session, it can be helpful to say, "I believe that this topic deserves more time and consideration than the few minutes we have left. Let's save it for our next time together."

If you or your client believe that the topic is important, you may wish to add another session some other time in the week. If a face-to-face session cannot be arranged, you may wish to hold a session over the phone (see Chapter 6).

When a Client Is Late for a Session

Give clients your back-line phone number and instructions to call if they will be late for a session. Occasional lateness and planned lateness should be totally acceptable. Nevertheless, when a client is late for a session, express concern and say, "I'm sorry we won't be able to have a full session today."

If a client does not show up and does not call, call him or her within the first ten minutes of the planned session. If necessary, leave a message on the client's answering machine. Depending on the circumstances, you can suggest finding a different time to meet, or formally recommend that treatment be terminated. If you intend to terminate treatment, make an attempt to talk with the client in person and send a follow-up letter (return receipt requested) explaining that you are terminating the therapy. Give the reasons why and list the names and phone numbers of three practitioners with whom the client may consult.

When a client is habitually late but pays on a regular basis, you can intermittently ask the client what benefit he or she is receiving from such an arrangement. Depending on the response, you may need to further investigate the meaning of lateness or include it as part of the acceptable process of psychotherapy. More than once a client has said to me, "Dr. Gold, I will pay you for the session, but will call you in advance if I'm not coming. However, when I do come and I am a little late, I would prefer not to view our sessions as another appointment I must keep."

Psychotherapy for many clients is psychologically and medically necessary. Many other clients want psychotherapy, though they do not suffer from serious mental disorders. They are interested in using the session and your services as a counselor.

Do You Charge a Client Who Misses a Session?

With certain exceptions, you should charge clients who miss a session. If an already-established client who has shown up and paid regularly misses one session, consider it an act of professional courtesy not to charge that person. For the most part, though, charge clients your full fee for any session missed. If you have a waiting list of clients, or current clients who wish an additional hour in a given week, and are able to schedule them in place of a client who misses a regular session, do not charge the client who was either a no-show or who canceled the appointment without a 24-hour notification.

'Tis the Season to Be Jolly

It is a popular myth that therapists receive a lot of emergency calls during the holiday season. Actually, expect to see less of your clients at this time. Clients who can afford to pay for a private practitioner can also afford vacations, and will typically reduce the number of clinical visits during the holiday season due to travel, festivities, and end-of-year business dealings. Starting at Thanksgiving and throughout the holidays, it has been my experience as an urban clinician that clients go through a "Friday-night syndrome," with January as their Monday morning. This syndrome occurs when the client puts a great deal of faith in holidays, weekends, or vacations to "correct" and "solve" their life problems. However, Monday morning, the last day of vacation, and the end of the holidays bring the client back to daily reality.

Should Clients Be Able to See a Clock?

With the exception of a psychoanalytic practice, clients should have the opportunity of gauging and weighing the time they wish to spend on various topics. This is not only in the clients' best interest, but serves the therapeutic process by making the clients aware of how they use their time and what its value is.

Place clocks so they face each of the walls of the office, in direct line of sight of you and your client. This way, either of you may look at a clock if you wish, giving you both the option of deciding to spend more or less time on a particular topic. Many therapists, depending on their theoretical orientation, disagree with this approach. I like having a clock in view because I feel the utilization of time and the focus of what is important in one's life is a central issue to everyone. One of the secondary gains of a psychotherapeutic session is effective time management and the establishment of self-regulating boundaries.

Une Ange Passe

I am sure you have heard clients lament, "I don't have anything to talk about today, so I feel I am wasting my time." Therapists also feel uncomfortable with long silences. The therapy session can be viewed as an exercise that helps people focus themselves in the presence of a guide. Sometimes, that focus is best done in silence.

Many years ago, a French client once told me about a colloquial French expression related to conversational silences: "une ange passe." Literally translated, it means "an angel is passing." My client explained that when an uncomfortable silence occurs, such as when everyone at a dinner table suddenly stops talking, the French break the tension by using this metaphor.

We should point out to our clients that the psychotherapeutic relationship is special. One aspect of its specialness is the acceptance of silence. This directly relates to Winacott's object relations concept of being alone in the presence of the mother. As therapists, we must help our clients re-frame the learned uncomfortableness of solitude in the presence of another human being. The psychotherapeutic process should be the guardian of another person's solitude. Most therapists need to learn this as much as their clients do.

Another metaphor for silence is the concept of fallow ground. The earth needs time to regenerate itself so that growth can begin anew. This conscientious use of land leads to greater productivity and makes for a plentiful harvest. The same holds true in psychotherapy. Through the psychotherapeutic relationship, we can teach our clients that resting with one's self is as important as working on one's self.

Doorknob Statements

"Doorknob statements" are remarks made by clients, and sometimes therapists, that provoke continued discussion and leave either party feeling a lack of closure. In interpersonal relationships, they often begin with the phrase "by the way." Aside from a concluding remark or gesture, a session should not end at the doorway, but while you and the client are still seated in your usual interface position.

Collecting your fee at the end of the hour may contribute to clients' addressing new topics or making doorknob statements. The following session format may help avoid this:

1. Greet the client in the consultation room.

2. Be seated and begin the therapy session.

3. Leave your seat and conduct economic business (exchange of checks, receipts, etc.).

4. Bid a final good-bye at the "escape door."

For those of you who do not have a secretary or receptionist to handle a client's arrival or departure, prepare a billing statement or receipt in advance.

It is therapeutically important to realize that most doorknob statements contain fodder for the next session. You can acknowledge this to a client with a statement such as "I would like to continue that train of thought in our next session," and then note the statement in your clinical records. This will aid both you and your client in dealing with anxiety-provoking material presented in a hit-and-run manner, as is typical of doorknob statements.

Taking Care of the Client by Staying in Touch

The handling of emergencies is a controversial area in psychotherapy. I inform my clients that if there is a genuine life-or-death situation, they should call 911 or their local emergency number. I also give them this advice for calling medical services, pointing out that people may lose valuable time for life-saving procedures trying to contact with their doctor first. After the emergency service has been called is the appropriate time to call the regular doctor or therapist.

One of the worst things you can do to a human being is to make them believe you can provide services that you can't. As a therapist, you should tell the truth even if it means losing those clients who want a clinician who is more readily available.

I believe that phone emergency issues are created by the therapist, not by the client. A clinician should clearly state his or her policy for handling serious emergencies during the first session with a client, and should return all calls within a reasonable period of time (no more than 24 hours). Clients who seem abusive with their phone calling are either not "working" during their therapy sessions or need more hours per week in therapy, or the clinician is underestimating the anxiety connected with a current event in the client's life.

While a person may need to talk to someone when a friend or loved one dies, I do not consider this a serious emergency. Even when a client you care about is grieving from a death, you must remain firm about your boundaries. If you have a gerontology practice or are dealing with the terminally ill, it will be especially important to establish boundaries and be clear about what you consider acceptable contact outside of therapy.

On the other hand, when a client is going through a difficult time, such as divorce, illness, or death in the family, touch base with that person on a daily basis. Take five minutes each day to make contact during the client's time of stress. I disagree with those who consider that this approach fosters a dependent relationship. Psychotherapy does build a genuine relationship between a client and therapist.

Touching base with a client as you would family and friends is also one of the strongest practice-builders I can recommend. When you have a client in distress, you take that person home with you—not like a worried mother but like a caring helper. A five-minute phone call tells the client that someone cares, and it will help put any fears you may have to rest. Clients need to know that we are there for them: the more we are there for them, the less chance a true emergency will arise.

Be present whenever possible, and to make it clear when you can't be. The process of letting go involves touching base. A clinician who knows a client is going through a horrendous situation and doesn't touch base is being irresponsible. When making calls to touch base, simply tell your client that you are calling between sessions and only have about five minutes to talk. This method is called "frontloading." It lets your client know up front what your situation is.

We all need a home base in our lives. The irony is that when we know we have it, we don't use it as much. Those who don't feel they have a home base have an urgent need to have at least a semblance of one on a regular basis. As psychotherapists we need to consider the client/therapist relationship as genuine.

Client Contact Outside of Sessions

The issue of client contact outside of a session has been a topic of debate since the beginning of psychotherapy. Most associations and state licensing boards reflect the psychoanalytic position that client/therapist contact outside of a session is unethical. In some states, it is illegal.

The case of the California therapist, who accepted professional housecleaning services as partial payment for therapy, is an example. The California state ethics committee ruled that this was a dual relationship and improper, and the impropriety was deemed serious enough for the practitioner's license to be revoked.

Dual relationships with clients are being viewed more conservatively all the time. If you anticipate having even the most casual association with a client outside of therapy, call your state association or licensing board anonymously and discuss the implications of that relationship.

Dual relationships can include knowing a person before he or she became a client, after the person leaves your practice (generally ending from two months to two years afterward), or while engaged with you in psychotherapy.

Examples of legitimate client contact include attending the funeral of a client's significant other, attending a graduation ceremony, attending the opening of a motion picture on which your client worked, and attending a celebration in honor of a client that is part of an achievement directly related to the therapy. I consider the above examples to be within the framework of the nonpsychoanalytic model and, at times, a necessary and supportive aspect of providing therapy.

These are not recommendations for what you should do. Indeed, sometimes transference on the part of the client would make attending such an event harmful to the therapeutic relationship. Make judgments on a client-by-client basis.

As professionals we have a sacred duty to fight for our clients' well-being at all costs. Sometimes that involves the bending or breaking of a particularly rigid code. So, although many of the laws and ethics under which we are required to operate were responses to harmful behaviors on the part of some psychotherapists, strict orthodoxy and rules do not apply to all situations. Times and people change, often more quickly than laws. I cannot, in good conscience, hide behind laws or ethics I consider, at times, hysterical reactions that produce unreasonable restrictions on my relationship with my client.

In my opinion, you cannot practice psychotherapy without occasionally stretching a boundary or breaking a rule. Neither you nor your clients are machines. I recommend the following procedures when you feel a conflict about what you should do:

1. Talk to your supervisor. I reserve one hour of didactic therapy per week to discuss my cases. For the continued supervision of your caseload, choose a "supervisor" who is senior in years, has a different theoretical orientation, and most importantly, is someone

you respect. I have found supervisors at conferences, at local universities, and through my own local grapevine. For any clinician working in a full-time private practice, supervision, although not required, is in my opinion a must.

2. Check with your state professional association or licensing board regarding possible consequences of your projected behavior.

3. Do what is best for your client and what you and your conscience can live with. These kinds of choices are faced by anyone genuinely engaged in a healing relationship with another human being.

Tips to Reduce Lawsuits

The following tips to minimize the risk of a lawsuit are from an article that appeared in the August 1990 issue of the American Psychological Association's monthly journal, *The Monitor*.

1. Keep your records accurate and up-to-date. John Murray, Chairman of the Insurance Trust, states: "documentation is so needed. It supports why the decision was made and under what circumstance." The article suggests that, by indicating the client's delusional system, records may be useful in helping prevent false allegations of sexual abuse.

2. Consult with colleagues whenever you are having a problem with a client. If you are later sued, such contact will demonstrate that you tried to solve the problem.

3. If you are in a supervisory capacity, make sure your trainees or interns carry their own malpractice insurance.

4. Stay away from dual relationships, especially business ventures.

5. Set the ground rules for confidentiality when therapy starts, especially if you are seeing adolescents. Make sure all waivers of confidentiality are in writing.

6. "Don't have sex with your clients. If you find yourself drawn to them romantically, immediately refer. But don't abandon them," advises Bruce Bennett, former Chief of the Insurance Trust. "If necessary, get help yourself."

8

Using Your Resources

This chapter includes professional consultations (medical, legal, institutional), support from other professions (accountants, business, and professional attorneys), and services provided by local and national associations. There is also a discussion of the "we treat" concept.

Visit your local technical bookstore to find many resources to aid you and your clients throughout your practice. It is extremely important to establish your own library and have it accessible during the hours of your practice. The following is a list of resources I use every week.

1. *Physicians Desk Reference*, Litton Industries (Mountvale, NJ), 1993

2. *The Merck Manual of Diagnosis and Therapy*, 16th edition, Keefer Lyght, Merck Sharp and Dohme Research Laboratories (Rahway, NJ), 1992

3. *Stedman's Medical Dictionary . . . Illustrated*, 25th edition, The Williams and Wilkins Company (Baltimore, MD), 1990

4. *Modern Synopsis of Comprehensive Textbook of Psychiatry V*, Harold Kaplan and Benjamin Sadock, Williams & Wilkins (Baltimore, MD), 1989

5. *The Psychiatric Interview in Clinical Practice*, Roger A. MacKinnon and Robert Michels, W.B. Saunders Company (New York), 1971

6. *Psychiatric Dictionary*, 5th edition, Robert Jean Campbell, Oxford University Press (New York), 1989

8. *DSM-III-R*, 3rd edition, revised, American Psychiatric Association (Washington, DC), 1987

9. *A Quick Reference to Diagnostic Criteria from DSM-III-R*, Robert L. Spitzer, American Psychiatric Association (Washington, DC), 1980

10. *DSM-III-R Casebook*, Robert L. Spitzer, American Psychiatric Association (Washington, DC), 1989

11. *The Psychotherapy Handbook*, Richie Herink, ed., The New American Library (New York), 1980

12. Newspapers, newsletters, magazines, and periodicals from the private sector as well as professional organizations (e.g., *The Monitor*, journal of the American Psychological Association, etc.)

Bibliotherapy

I believe books can significantly aid clients in their healing process, and over the years I have recommended thousands of books to clients. In the self-help and psychology sections of your local bookstore, you will find many books to benefit both you and your client. You can also recommend motion pictures, videos, songs, literary works, poetry, and art as ways for clients to connect with images and ideas that will help clarify their problems and dilemmas.

Many excellent books have recently been published on the new masculinity, including works by Robert Bly, Joseph Campbell, and Sam Keen. However, to a client struggling with issues related to the masculine psyche, you can also recommend reading the classic *Zorba the Greek*.

The leader of a workshop on human sexuality suggested that when discussing sexuality with younger children or adolescents, clinicians should use books without photographs of genitalia or delivery. This leader felt that books with such photographs may make too much of an impression on younger clients, as these clients may compare their genitals with those in the photographs. It was recommended that clinicians find books with illustrations rather than photographs. In sum, the suggestion was to keep the clinical experience as aesthetically pleasing and nonthreatening as possible.

Likewise, literature may allow a client distance sometimes not afforded by a book more clinical in nature. *Fear of Flying* can be as effective in bibliotherapy as *The Wounded Woman*. A video of *To Kill a Mockingbird* may teach more about parenting than clinical parenting texts. When dealing with sexual dysfunction, try having clients read National Lampoon's spoof of *The Joy of Sex*, entitled *The Job of Sex*. People who can laugh with one another have a greater chance of overcoming sexual dysfunction than people who only "study" sexuality together.

Testing Services

As a clinician, you may prefer to do your own psychological or neurological testing. As a sole practitioner, I have found that using a testing service is a better use of my time and money than administering and hand scoring my own MMPIs (Minnesota Multiphasic Personality Inventories) or using a database program to score them.

There are many testing services, including Caldwell Reports, Western Psychological Services, and Minnesota Testing Services. These services all deliver excellent, thorough, narrative reports to the private practitioner. Western Psychological Services provides more clinical scales, is relatively inexpensive, and is helpful in interpreting scores.

Inpatient/Outpatient Facilities

Even if your practice consists mainly of clients suffering from psychoneurotic disorders rarely requiring hospitalization, you may find that your clients perceive you as the person to call in an emergency requiring the hospitalization of a family member or friend. Therefore, it makes sense to maintain relationships with admitting physicians at both private and state mental institutions within a 50-mile radius of your office.

Familiarize yourself with the involuntary commitment laws, and establish protocols for whom to call and which agency to contact in urgent situations. Call your state association, and the state and local associations of other disciplines, for information and assistance relating to involuntary commitment, voluntary hospitalizations, medication evaluations, and other urgent clinical issues that may arise.

Remember that public and private hospitals want your business. Investigate voluntary and involuntary hospital settings and their policies, perhaps over lunch with the hospital's marketing representative. Though they tend to present a picture that is a little too rosy, marketing people can be helpful regarding services and costs within (or beyond) the scope of your practice. I also recommend that you ask whether or not you would be allowed to maintain appropriate contact with your client during a hospital stay.

Workshops

Attending workshops is similar to going on first dates. Neither usually fulfills your highest expectations or your worst fears. The greatest benefits of workshops are networking with other professionals; finding placements for special-problem clients; and learning about new techniques, reporting laws, rules and regulations, and ways of stimulating client traffic; and they are a great excuse to have a vacation in a city you may not have visited had the trip not been tax-deductible. Workshops are places where we can get some of Maslow's needs met while getting a tax break.

Local and National Associations

Local and national associations are becoming political action committees vying for shares of the mental health market. Mental health practitioners from various disciplines are represented by separate state and national organizations that are often adversarial. For example, many psychiatrists do not want psychologists to have admitting privileges in hospitals. And some state associations fight for legislation to exclude practitioners with other credentials from receiving insurance reimbursements from both the private and public sectors.

These associations depend on your dollars to continue these battles and pay their salaries. As a clinician, you should expect to receive services in return for your annual dues. Many associations offer such services as newsletters, research literature, referrals, and limited legal and financial counseling. Over the years, the associations you belong to can be extremely helpful to you. Get what you pay for and use your affiliations!

Medical, Institutional, and Legal Consultations

Medical Consultations

Many emotional problems have a medical concomitant cause and vice versa. After you have obtained proper release of confidential information forms, it will sometimes be necessary to consult with clients' medical providers. A few minutes on the phone with a medical provider can yield information that you will find significant and revealing. Fill out a professional consultation form while talking with a consultant (see Clinical Consultation form on page 91).

Begin your conversation by introducing yourself and informing the physician that you are treating one of his or her patients. Explain that you have asked the client when his or her last complete physical was and what the results were.

You will find that most doctors are responsive if you offer to aid in serving their patients. Medical practitioners are more cognizant of psychological factors and more willing to consult with psychotherapists than they were years ago.

Often a physician will be surprised to find out that a patient has entered psychotherapy. Most of the time you will get a positive reaction from the physician. Medical doctors do not make money by talking to their patients; they make money by performing procedures. Since therapists are paid to listen to clients at length, they relieve medical doctors of having to spend time talking with their patients.

Institutional Consultations

Institutional consultations can be frustrating. Talking to school counselors and other professionals who deliver counseling services has proved to me to be more beneficial than talking to bureaucrats who steadfastly enforce a particular system, such as some probation and parole officers. On the other hand, I do not envy their roles or caseloads.

When you are dealing with institutional settings and the people who can access information about you and your client, I cannot suggest strongly enough that you personalize your contact with them. After an initial phone consultation, send them your card or a thank-you note. Write a quick letter to their supervisor saying how much you appreciate their service. With the enormity of cutbacks in the public sector today, civil servants must be handled with the care we wish for ourselves.

CLINICAL CONSULTATIONS

CLIENT'S NAME:		CLIENT'S ID NO.	DATE:

Date:	Consultant's Name:		Profession:
	Address:		
	Telephone:		
	Client's Release of Confidentiality signed:		Date:
PURPOSE OF CONSULT ☐ MEDICAL ☐ PSYCHIATRIC ☐ LEGAL ☐ TESTING ☐ SCHOOL ☐ OTHER	**COMMENTS:**		

Date:	Consultant's Name:		Profession:
	Address:		
	Telephone:		
	Client's Release of Confidentiality signed:		Date:
PURPOSE OF CONSULT ☐ MEDICAL ☐ PSYCHIATRIC ☐ LEGAL ☐ TESTING ☐ SCHOOL ☐ OTHER	**COMMENTS:**		

Date:	Consultant's Name:		Profession:
	Address:		
	Telephone:		
	Client's Release of Confidentiality signed:		Date:
PURPOSE OF CONSULT ☐ MEDICAL ☐ PSYCHIATRIC ☐ LEGAL ☐ TESTING ☐ SCHOOL ☐ OTHER	**COMMENTS:**		

Legal Consultations

A client's litigation can be one of the most frightening things to a clinician (beginning or experienced) who is not familiar with forensic psychology. Usually, a clinician will receive a subpoena duces tecum, which essentially requests that all records be provided either at a deposition or for reproduction at the request of an attorney. Be familiar with the laws of your state pertaining to confidentiality and privilege. Your state association can help you understand subpoenas and legal requests. It is important for a clinician, with proper releases, to speak to a client's attorney regarding legal requests.

There are, in fact, subpoenas that can be acknowledged, ignored, or refused. To achieve the best results for your client, consult with your client's legal counsel. Certain standard clichés, such as "emotional pain and suffering," frequently used in the filing of lawsuits, may or may not apply to the lawsuit in which your client is involved. For example, a client may not be aware that the attorney representing him in a case involving whiplash from an auto accident has included claims of "emotional pain and suffering" in the lawsuit.

In California, suing someone for emotional suffering of any kind automatically waives the privilege and confidentiality of the plaintiff's psychotherapeutic records, giving the defendant's representatives the right to view all of them. This is because the person being sued has a right to investigate the client's mental state, including both preexisting conditions and conditions presently being treated.

You can make it a standard of practice to ask your clients during the initial interview if, to their knowledge, anything you will discuss may be used in legal proceedings. You can also ask clients to inform you whenever they file a lawsuit against someone so you can discuss confidentiality and privilege pertaining to your therapeutic relationship. I inform my clients that my records can be subpoenaed under certain circumstances. In California, if a client is involved in a traffic accident and sues the other party to the accident, the attorney often includes in the lawsuit a request for monies related to mental and emotional pain and suffering. In such circumstances, case law demands that the clinician release information relating to the client's mental status prior to, during, and after the accident.

Attorneys are used to generating paperwork and can be of assistance if you are asked to submit a report. Attorneys also know what aspect of a report is most helpful to emphasize on your client's behalf. The summary of the report is often the only thing ever read by a hearing officer or judge. Ask your client's legal counsel what points should be emphasized in a summary relating to the particular case. For example, many attorneys have asked me to indicate the cost of future therapy for their clients. Ordinarily, this is something I would not have thought to include in a summary report.

Accountants and Attorneys

You can save yourself a lot of worry by consulting with an accountant familiar with tax laws relating to psychotherapists, and with an attorney acquainted with both the business and professional aspects of therapeutic practice. It is barely possible to run a practice and still keep current on the new clinical issues that arise every day; by meeting with an accountant and an attorney with the above qualifications and experience, you will not only rest easier, but will feel up-to-date on other issues that can seriously affect your practice. It is part of their job to follow new developments you may not have time to follow.

If you do not have an accountant or attorney familiar with private business, ask other clinicians and your local and state associations for referrals. Professionals from other professions who specialize in aiding people in psychology sometimes advertise in psychology journals. When you contact a professional for legal or accounting services, request a resume and the names of other clients you can contact to assess the professional's competence in your area of practice.

It pays to consult with your accountant before setting up your bookkeeping system. With an accountant's aid, you can devise a simple system that will tell you at a glance your accounts payable and your accounts receivable, and what accounting you need to do at any given time.

A few hundred dollars of prevention is worth thousands of dollars and grief in the cure! Meeting with a business and professions attorney once a year is a great way to keep informed about the attitudes of the legal system in relation to your clinical work. These professionals tend to know what legal and ethical considerations are the most sensitive, and their advice can aid you in making on-the-spot clinical responses that reflect the climate of the times. You may wish to continue practicing as you always have, though some methods of practice may pose a danger to your license; but you will be making an informed decision. An example of this situation is the highly publicized and scrutinized issue of touching between therapist and client. The current ethics seem to follow a strict psychoanalytic bias (i.e., any touching is bad). A humanist, however, may believe it is important to continue practicing nonsexual, non-violational touching or hugging. By consulting with a business and professions attorney, you will know the current risks attendant on your decision.

The "We Treat" Policy

The "we treat" policy means feeling confident that, if there is relief or cure possible for your client's pain, you can find it *or* find a resource for it. Over the past 25 years I have developed a network of clinicians and professionals working in allied fields; this network provides me with a professional safety net when I devise a treatment plan for my clients. A sensitive, effective therapist does not practice in a vacuum, and this perspective is part and parcel of the "we treat" concept.

Humility and the knowledge that all of us need the aid of others are prerequisites to being a competent psychotherapist and human being. Although as a psychotherapist I sometimes feel as though I am alone on an island, the truth is that there are many islands to keep in view, to communicate and consult with, and to ask our clients to visit. The concept of "we treat" leaves me feeling lighter and better able to treat my clients with competency and fairness.

It is important to remember when consulting another professional for personal support or professional feedback to maintain your clients' confidentiality. This can be done either by obtaining a signed release from your client allowing you to talk with another professional regarding the therapy, or by disguising your client's identity in your conversations.

Group Therapy

I believe group therapy is a great form of adjunctive therapy for people who wish to socialize and have positive mirroring. During the 11 years that I conducted encounter groups, I found that people benefited from the socialization process but were not receiving focused psychotherapy. People in need of therapy should not seek group therapy.

I rarely send anyone to a nonspecific group, but have recommended specifically oriented groups that to clients. Good examples of such groups are an assertiveness training group that reviews behaviors designed for assertiveness training, and all-male or -female support groups.

If you are starting a therapy group today, pick a hot topic (e.g., based on a best-selling book like *Codependent No More*), and then do direct-market advertising. Through target-market identification, you will be able to advertise inexpensively. One of my business associates, for example, started a women's professional group and advertised in the "B'nai Brith Messenger," which specifically targets single Jewish females. Since advertising that she leads focus groups, this clinician now runs a very successful private practice.

Twelve-Step Programs

Twelve-step programs are beneficial because the group's participants welcome each person's shame, and there is no cross talk. Someone shares his or her story, and no one has anything to gain except wellness.

Over the years, there have been fears voiced about Twelve-step programs having bad economic effects on private practices. I do not believe this to be true. I think Twelve-step programs lead people in need of psychotherapy to therapists. I am delighted these programs exist and are accessible to those who need them. The fourth step, which requires a rigorous moral inventory of oneself, usually leads people into psychotherapy, or at least to an interest in further self-exploration.

Most municipalities have several different Twelve-step programs. By contacting your city, county, or state alcoholism council, you can receive excellent information on how to help your clients begin their work in a Twelve-step program. The local alcoholism council will often have a list of hotlines and other support groups in your area.

Your Support Network

Private practice can be lonely. We are not permitted, ethically, to share our work as other people can. We hear and are exposed to scenarios that can sicken, anger, and frighten us. We need someone with whom we can continuously confide and consult.

Take a minute right now to close your eyes and think of all of the professional contacts you have needed in order to open your private practice or run it for any number of years. Picture the faces of those people who support your work.

Listen to your current clients' remarks about other professionals who treat them, and ask your clients to bring you the business cards of these others. Contact these and other professionals recommended by colleagues, mentors, or friends, and suggest a lunch. Meeting with colleagues will help you establish professional confidantes, expand your referral network, and exchange information that influences your practice. When meeting with them, try to determine the following:

1. How do their services fit into the scope of your practice?

2. How does your practice fit into the scope of their profession?

3. What is their availability and fee structure?

4. What are their special interests, hobbies, and professional specialties?

5. What is their perception of the people with whom they work?

6. What is their prognosis of the future of their profession?

7. What is their personal and professional philosophy?

8. Who are other colleagues they would refer someone to if they were too busy or could not accept the fees your clients could pay?

9. What are their perceptions of you and how you might be useful to them and their clientele?

10. Do you like them?

You will still have your dark and lonely times, but keep sight of the fact that there are many of us there to support and aid you and your clients in the search for well-being. We need one another.

9

The Therapist's Wastebasket: Sorry, It's a Dirty Job...

How Long Should the Therapy Process Last?

When I entered therapy in the mid-1970s with a Jungian analyst, I asked him at our fourth or fifth session how long the therapeutic process would take. I will never forget his response: "Michael, I have taught you everything there is to know. It will take you about 20 years to hear it."

The answer to how long therapy should last is: it depends.

The consensus among psychotherapy practitioners is that there seems to be more than one breaking point in the psychotherapeutic process. Whether it is in their best interests or not, most clients seem to terminate their therapy according to this time frame:

1. After four to six weeks

2. After six months

3. After two years

4. Never

5. Any combination of the first four, with intermittent visits, according to individual adjustment reactions

Time frames relating to the beginning and end of therapy can be discussed at the beginning of therapy, during therapy, or when a client feels the end is near. With the advent of managed care, many clients will be anxiously aware of how many sessions their insurance will allow for outpatient psychotherapy. Be prepared for more and more "how long will this take?" questions.

Handling Disagreements with Clients

Let your clients know up front that you want to know if they disagree with you or if you have made a mistake. If the client does not feel comfortable explaining what happened face-to-face, ask the client to telephone instead. Make it clear that no matter how angry the client is, you need help in understanding your faux pas and thus avoiding hurting another client in the same way. Keeping the lines of communication open is very important.

Over the years, my clients have responded in many ways to what they have perceived as clinical errors. Some have written me, some have called, and some have stopped their therapy with me. When this happens I try to contact the client and discuss the reasons. The information I have received from these discussions has often been helpful in my work with other clients. Also, great therapy has sometimes gone on after a client and I have *not* been able to reach an agreement.

Never be afraid of losing a client. For every client you lose, you can gain ten. Encourage clients to seek information from other experts. They will remember you as a giver and gain confidence in you as an honest practitioner. If clients have confidence in you but know you cannot help them in therapy, making a few phone calls will show that you have a vast array of resources you are willing to call upon for help. This is the benchmark of an ethical practitioner and a good practice-builder.

The one commandment of all private practices is: "Thou shalt not do greater damage than has already been done."

"Wheel Hitters"

I have occasionally felt it necessary to call a client after experiencing a "wheel hitter" in my car on the way home from work. I suddenly realize that there is unfinished business left over from a session, and react by hitting the steering wheel of my car.

When I call the client, I say that I have leftover thoughts and feelings from our session and ask if the client feels the same. I handle a "wheel hitters" in this way because I don't want to carry around excess baggage, and because I encourage my clients to be open and honest with me. My clients are invited to call me if they experience similar feelings.

Some clinicians disagree with this practice, feeling that such follow-up contact introduces too much of a countertransference response. In such a situation, they might suggest that therapists talk only to their supervisors, and wait to discuss it with the client until he or she brings up the issue in a future session.

Abusive Clients

Clients with narcissistic personality disorders or aggressive or nonaggressive antisocial personality disorders are often abusive and malevolent. Obsessive/compulsives and paranoids may have periods when they don't do a bad job on your head either! Clients with borderline personality disorders and paranoid schizophrenic disorders also abuse therapists, but with less regularity.

Common behaviors of abusive clients include:

- showing up late for appointments
- missing appointments without appropriate notification
- failing to comply with agreed-upon economic arrangements (not paying for sessions)
- excessive and inappropriate use of phone contacts
- abusing clerical personnel or other patients while in the waiting room
- making threatening insinuations or gestures relating to bodily harm
- making threatening insinuations relating to lawsuits directed at the clinician

Our profession tends to tolerate and use a person's anger and rage in the psychotherapeutic process, but we still have a responsibility to ourselves and others to protect everyone concerned from abusive, dangerous behavior.

Borderline narcissistic clients may endanger a therapist's license by making sexual advances; they need to be confronted about their abusive behavior. While recent emphasis has been placed on therapists being sexually abusive, the opposite can also be true.

Try to identify any disorder or abuse from a client within the first four trial consultations. As therapists, we have a responsibility not to harm our clients. If you refer these types of clients, send them to a therapist willing to treat them, or to a specialized clinician.

I cannot stress enough the importance of having a referral list of your own. It is one of the most valuable services you can offer as you build your private practice. Psychotherapy is not a point-of-purchase commodity. You cannot be available to all those who want your services.

Clients Who Don't Pay

Another example of abuse is not paying for a session. One way to handle a client who does not pay is to end the relationship. Period.

Sometimes, however, a therapist may not be aware that a client has no intention of paying. Some clients may come to therapy presenting an indirect problem, such as a problem with their spouse, rather than what may be a real problem, such as sociopathic behavior or substance abuse. Others may be court-ordered into therapy, but have no desire for therapeutic treatment and they may not inform you of the situation. Because the therapy may not address their core problem, or because they want to use the money for drugs, or simply because they don't feel they should have therapy, these clients may avoid paying for services, refuse to pay for services, or "disappear" without paying. Do not regret such situations—they happen to everyone; but be aware they do exist.

Unless you have made a special agreement because a client is experiencing economic hardship, clients should pay within one month of service. Do not abandon a client who is in financial difficulties, but if a client does not pay for malevolent reasons, end the relationship.

How to End a Relationship with a Client

Based on experience, I am candid with certain clients who are substance abusers, telling them that I feel psychotherapy is a waste of time and that a Twelve-step program might be more effective for them. In my practice, I have seen these types of clients suffer neurological as well as psychological damage as a result of substance abuse.

Therapists have an enormous responsibility not to collude with these clients. A therapist's job is to break good news, not to be a coroner. Psychotherapy is a waste of everyone's time when the client is clearly on a self-induced deathbed. However, if the substance abuser is willing to be *in* therapy and not just *going to* therapy, as a psychotherapist I am always delighted to seem them.

If you have a client that you cannot treat for whatever reason—lack of time, lack of experience with the disorder, your own inappropriate countertransferences to people suffering from specific disorders—use the concept of "we treat" discussed in Chapter 8. Try to refer these clients to clinicians or agencies that are better able to provide the care they need. However, contact the clinicians or agencies in advance to inform them of your diagnosis and the difficulties you had in treating the client, either after receiving your client's permission or by not identifying the client.

Client dumping is not only unethical, it is abusive—to the client and to your colleagues. One clinician's client is another clinician's grief. By respecting both the client and your colleagues, you will, with few exceptions, be able to match clients who are difficult for you to treat with appropriate clinicians.

The Last Session

The question of how to terminate a client's therapy is a never-ending discussion. Depending on your theoretical background, you have been or are being trained to handle termination sessions in various ways. There are many books on this aspect of the therapeutic process. Most of these include style and content on terminating a client. That is not the focus of this section.

Something I have done for many years that has proved fruitful is to inform the client that the last session is "on the house." Offering a free final session encourages clients who would otherwise avoid termination procedures to attend. Having personally experienced an abrupt ending of psychotherapy, I feel it is in the service of my current and future clients to understand the nature and reasons for termination. Discussing this with clients candidly allows me to make adjustments in the way I practice towards certain clients as well as informs me what practices and procedures I should continue.

When possible, I ask the client to schedule an appointment six months after the termination session. At the six-month point, I will ask the client to keep in touch with me on a yearly basis, explaining that much of the processing that goes on in therapy will surface later and is useful long after the therapy terminates.

During the last session, I tell clients that it is helpful to me as a practitioner to know what they remember as most useful or hurtful during the time we spent together.

Sometimes my clients move great distances, and I request that they drop me a line or give me a call every six months and then once a year for five years. Over the years, about 30% of my clientele have contacted me over that five-year period. I refer to these calls as mental health checkups and do not charge for this service. They help me assess my psychotherapeutic process, which includes long-term results.

I understand that some of you may consider this a countertransference need on my part. It may be, but it is the only method I can think of that gives me feedback over an extended period of time. If your philosophical orientation will accept this methodology, I highly recommend it.

As clinicians, we tend to forget that we need to research our methodology and techniques. If you have other suggestions for accomplishing this task, please send a letter to me in care of my publisher. I would love to find new and better ways of practicing all aspects of my psychotherapy and would credit you with ideas in future editions of this book.

Today, there is a certain feeling, perhaps adopted from insurance companies, as to how long "it" (psychotherapy) should last. With so many diagnoses found in the DSM-III-R, there are times when I wonder if sessions should be paid for by any outside agency. Then again, as a believer in socialized medicine, I feel a system should be implemented whereby all citizens who need treatment get it and all therapists who need money earn it.

10

Terminating Your Practice

This chapter looks at topics related to terminating your practice, whether it is because you are relocating, selling, or closing up shop altogether.

Clinicians terminate their practice for different reasons. They may move to another clinic or another city, retire, sell their practice, or significantly change their availability and hours of practice. They may suffer a long-term illness, or die.

I use the word *terminate* because that is how clients experience the situation. Just as you cannot predict your clients' futures, neither can you predict your own future. It is our responsibility as therapists to plan with care the opening, development, and running of our practice. We also have a professional responsibility to plan for the ending of our practice with equal care and to help our clients accept it whenever we can.

As you know, many clients demonstrate some form of anger when their therapist returns from an extended holiday. Depending on the client, the diagnosis, the transference, and the particular stage of therapy the person is in, the reactions and behavior will differ.

Try to develop policies for handling temporary as well as permanent separations between your and your clients, before you need them. For example, during your internship, inform clients about the length of your internship and the options they will have when the internship has ended. Decide whether you want to address this issue verbally with individual clients or to include it in the introductory packet of information given to the client at the beginning of the psychotherapeutic process. If you are with a clinic, they may have their own policies regarding how to deal with separations.

Over the years, I have experienced the death of my therapist, my family physician, and my internist. I have used these experiences in forming my own methods for dealing with separations.

The psychotherapist informed me at the beginning of our relationship that he had a terminal illness and that his life expectancy was one to three years. Four weeks before he died, as his health worsened, we began discussing "our parting." Although his death caused me to feel profound sadness, it seemed natural. Because I was prepared by him, I was able to make choices, and when I look back upon our relationship, his death is not the focus of my memories.

My family doctor of 41 years developed a serious heart condition 10 years before his death. I was informed that he would be reducing his hours and not taking new patients, but would continue his practice. He was not a verbal man, but my knowledge of his disease enabled me to continue our relationship with appropriate defenses, and helped me go through the sadness of his death.

My internist of 21 years killed himself. I dropped in for a visit and found a crowd of people crying in the waiting room. He had shared his psychological turmoil with me over the years, and I knew that his bipolar illness might someday lead to his untimely death. But I saw him the week before he took his life: we spoke for about half an hour and arranged to meet the following week. To this day his death has left me, at times, numb and questioning. Suicide has been sardonically referred to as "hanging your skeleton in another person's closet." His skeleton still hangs in my closet.

Based on my experiences with the loss of clinicians who were important to me, and on discussions of this issue with colleagues, I have formulated the following rules.

1. If you know you are going to terminate your practice because of illness, change of venue, change of careers, or retirement, it is your responsibility, whenever possible, to inform your clients at least one year in advance.

2. Give your clients the names of other clinicians whom you respect and trust as alternative therapists.

3. Discuss the disposition of your clinical records with your clients, and accommodate their wishes to the fullest possible extent.

4. Make provisions with colleagues regarding your files, and give them written permission to "seize" your records and clinical notations. Check state laws and association ethics regarding the dis-

position of your records. A business and professions attorney can help you draw up a simple document that will allow your colleagues to dispose of and disperse your records legally and ethically.

If we are to believe the modern writings of Alice Miller, Heinz Kohut, and Arno Gruen, we must face the issue of leaving our practices voluntarily or involuntarily as it relates to client abandonment. Most of us, clients as well as therapists, have strong conscious and unconscious reactions to abandonment.

In all primate species, individuals who are abandoned can die as a result. This is a practical reality for the species, as well as a result of narcissistic wounding. As you know, we all tend to confuse rejection with abandonment, reacting similarly to them emotionally. Our feelings relating to abandonment are rage, loss, depression, sadness, loss of hope or faith, and grief. As psychotherapists, we have a moral responsibility to account for those feelings in our clients, which can result from our planned leaving or sudden death, by making responsible arrangements.

Selling Your Practice

When selling your practice, consider the following questions:

1. How much does your practice make? What is your net income from it? What is the gross income? What is your operating cost—what does it basically cost to run your practice? Subtract the operating cost from the gross income to find the net income.

2. What is the current state of your treatment community? By treatment community, I mean current clients plus over all billable hours; other clinicians who refer clients to you; former clients who remain in touch or continue to refer clients to you; and social agencies, schools, and other regular referral sources for your practice.

3. If you are selling your practice lock, stock, and barrel, how much did you pay for your office furniture, appliances, testing materials, computers, computer materials, and library?

4. Have some of the above items increased or decreased in value over the years? If so, by how much? What are their current values, considering depreciation?

5. Compare your current rent with that in other, comparable offices. Is it high, low, or average?

6. Do you have an exceptionally good lease?

7. Do you have an unusually good landlord?

8. Is your office located in an area that could increase the business of a future clinician? The most difficult aspect to evaluate in terms of establishing a selling price is what is called good will. If you have been practicing at the same location for a long time, your entire treatment community, especially past and present clients, will have positive associations with that location. This is true even if many of your clients call for help in selecting other practitioners of the healing arts, and not only for professional consultations.

The biggest question on the mind of a person who is considering whether to purchase your practice is whether or not your current clientele will continue to see you rather than refer to a new clinician. To help you, your clients, and the clinician buying your practice adjust, you may wish to phase in the new clinician by starting groups run by both of you or having sessions conjointly attended by you and your new associate.

Moving Your Practice

You may decide to move from the area in which your practice is established for a variety of good reasons. A change in your health may require a change of climate. You may discover that you need to express yourself through a hobby or another profession rather than by practicing psychotherapy. Sometimes you just need a sabbatical.

We cannot predict our futures any more than our clients can.

Keeping this in mind, consider the following ideas: stay in touch with clinicians who practice or live in a location that is convenient for your clients. Besides locale, look for psychotherapists to whom you would go for treatment. Be on the lookout for therapists who practice and believe as you do, as well as for competent and loving people who practice other forms of psychotherapy.

As you locate practitioners for consultation on other topics (the "we treat" policy), look particularly for colleagues who know how to handle loss, anger, regret, resentment, sadness, depression, and anxiety, for yourself as well as your clients. Many of these feelings will surface in you when you decide to terminate, sell, or move your practice.

11

The Politics of Psychotherapy

Spinoza said, "There is no such thing as a nonpolitical man." In this chapter, I have tried to demonstrate that it is extremely difficult, at times, to separate serious clinical considerations from the political economic system.

What Is the Best Form of Therapy?

Since the first shamanistic healing took place, probably during the Paleolithic era, students and professionals have been sitting around caves and classrooms asking the following questions: What is the best form of therapy? What makes a good therapist? Does therapy really help? What is the nature of the therapist-client relationship? We are still asking these questions today, and things don't look good for our finding the answers any time soon.

Like any other profession, ours is influenced by the political climate of our time. Psychotherapy has gone through, is going through, and will go through many changes. In the DSM-III, I was amused to find it states if a woman can't have an orgasm during intromission, she could be diagnosed as anorgasmic. However, if a man cannot have an orgasm during intromission, he is undiagnosable. After political and feminist input, this criteria for anorgasmia was dropped. Now, in the DSM-III-R, if a man cannot have an orgasm during intromission, he is considered anorgasmic. Ahhh . . . the politics of mental illness.

As in national politics, the "hot" issues in our field are constantly changing. I read in journals of national psychotherapeutic organizations that ethics are a hot topic now, particularly concerning the nature of dual relationships. Other hot topics include what to report, who to report, who to report it to, and when to report.

In fact, reporting has become a hot topic in other fields as well. There is legislation now that makes it criminal not to report certain things, such as suspected child abuse. There are even advertisements exhorting us to report our neighbors for workers' compensation fraud, excessive vehicle emissions, and unsafe driving. I am extremely concerned that law has replaced ethics and that principles have replaced people.

When Allende was deposed from Chile, the new totalitarian regime executed university professors and psychologists first. Psychotherapy has the potential to change people's lives, and to help people see the truth in spite of the pain that may accompany it.

When we aid clients by "teaching them about their dysfunctional family," whether we like it or not, we change their "politics of experience."

When we facilitate clients' getting out of their own way, they become more productive. That productivity sometimes results in major life-changes like leaving their families, their jobs, and in some cases, their country.

If we are indeed "agents of change," we must accept the responsibility that we do anxiety-provoking and sometimes dangerous things.

Your challenge as a clinician will not come from which form of therapy you use in a given situation; it will come from your daily decisions about what is in your client's best interests, and following through even if it causes you anxiety.

I believe we are allowing too many others dictate the ethics of psychotherapy. We are sacrificing our clients' well-being to profit from insurance companies, letting them dictate the length of the therapeutic process by setting limits to payment. Attorneys, through the legal system, are determining the kinds and qualities of relationships needed to practice in the healing arts. The legislature's mandatory reporting acts are, in many cases, causing greater harm than they alleviate.

We must fight for our civil rights as well as those of our clients. We must increase and welcome the most extreme points of view relating to diagnosis and treatment. We must support laboratory and clinical research of the diseases we treat and look at what role we should play in their treatment. We must not lose that most fundamental tool in the process of being human: curiosity.

We must distrust simple answers to complex questions. If we lose the curious nature of our profession, we lose the right to have one.

Finally, I believe there is increased governmental, insurance company, and public service agency intrusion into the privacy and confidentiality necessary for human beings to express themselves openly and honestly. Harmful legal precedents, based on the extreme behaviors of a very few psychotherapists, have interfered in the therapeutic process and, in some cases, damaged clients. As we pollute our environment, we sanitize our relationships, refusing to recognize that being intimate with people is, by nature, messy.

Trendy Diagnoses and Treatments

Our profession is greatly influenced by and reactive to the political, economic, and social trends that are continuously advertised and are a way of life for our clients as well as ourselves. Self-help groups and seminars, ranging from Tony Robbins'"inspirational" lectures and activities to John Bradshaw's intensive workshops, have become a way of life. These speakers, along with the new "media shrinks," from Sonya Friedman to David Viscott, have become a part of our clients' psychological information bank. All of these are merely the latest in the chain of psychotherapy trends.

In the late sixties and early seventies, there was a great emphasis on humanistic/existential psychology. Balancing this, behavioral therapy was taking hold of the clinical world. With the publication of Johnson and Masters' work, *Human Sexual Inadequacy*, and the introduction of their technique of sensate focus, behaviorism was associated with a more liberal attitude.

Psychopharmacology, which had always been present in the treatment of psychotic disorders, began to be more widespread in the mid to late seventies with the introduction of the new long-acting antidepressant and antianxiety medications.

The trendy diagnoses that began in the mid to late sixties and early seventies emphasized posttraumatic stress disorder, drug rehabilitation, and milieu therapy. Beginning in the seventies, many of our clients came to us with diseases their physicians were unable to cure: hypoglycemia, PMS, chronic fatigue syndrome, and viruses such as herpes and Epstein-Barr. These and other medical diagnoses have begun seeking psychological comfort.

In the eighties, we saw the emergence of neo-Freudian analysis, using techniques and concepts from Heinz Kohut, Margaret Mahler, and Alice Miller. This turned the focus of analytic psychotherapy from "born with" drives to object relations. Along with the Christian fundamentalist movement that gained power during the Reagan and Bush administrations, a counterbalancing "spiritual" form of psychotherapy, called *transpersonal psychotherapy*, was emerging. Transpersonal psychotherapy recalls and repopularizes the works of Jung and the mythological works exemplified by Joseph Campbell, Robert Bly, and Sam Keen.

As an era of obsessiveness, compulsiveness, anxiety, and depression, the eighties saw the emergence of Xanax and Prozac. The severe economic recession resulted in an increase in paranoid, as well as self-flagellating, thought processes and behaviors.

As the romantic notion of marriage became pervasive in our society in the thirties and forties, so the romantic notion of "instant cure" psychotherapy has become part of our clients' expectations. Today we face a generation that has come to expect the best, sees greed as good, and gives logical explanations for its racism or ethnocentrism. On top of this, partly because of reduced benefits from insurance companies for outpatient treatment, additional pressures of time and money have entered the treatment room.

Some of the treatments and diagnoses I have shared with you have already faded. Some have lasted longer than expected. Some will be classic, and some will be chronic.

The DSM-IV: Political and Economic Implications

The DSM-IV is upon us. As of this writing, field tests, trials, and committee meetings are taking place so that the DSM-IV and all of its changes will be ready for publication in the spring of 1994. There is a faction of the American Psychiatric Association that wishes to delay the publication of the DSM-IV until 1998. They feel that there has not been enough time to institute the diagnostic changes recommended by the DSM-IV committees. They also believe that diagnostic manuals should be published with a minimum of 10 years' separation to allow for clinical trials over an extended period of time. In the Spring of 1993, however, the APA voted to release the DSM-IV in 1994.

The DSM-IV and the ICD-10 are to be produced in cooperation with the World Health Organization as part of a treaty obligation between the WHO and the United States. The idea behind this joint publication is to standardize reporting nomenclature as well as the coding system, which will be altogether different from that in the DSM-III-R. The American Psychiatric Association, in its book *DSM-IV Options Book: Work In Pro-*

gress (1991), has set up "five to ten different sites with approximately 100 subjects at each site" to field test the diagnostic changes and additions they are considering in the DSM-IV. According to this book, the APA is considering adding as many as 40 new categories and sections, as well as changing the coding system from the five-digit numerical system in the DSM-III-R to the single letter and four numbers of the ICD-10 coding system. All new diagnoses will be preceded by the letter F.

In addition to the changes in categories and coding, there are recommendations to eliminate or revise the current five-axis diagnostic system. From the original recommendations, it seems that a great number of clinicians believe that Axis IV and Axis V should be revised to include more subtle subcategories. As a reminder, Axis IV is the Psychosocial Stressor Scale (0–6), and Axis V is the Global Assessment of Functioning Scale (1–90) for the client's current level of functioning and his or her highest level of functioning in the past year. It appears that the objections, especially to Axis V, have to do with clinicians feeling limited by not being able to break down the different areas of functioning into different axes or sub-axes. As an example, one of the recommendations is to exchange the Axis V GAF Scale for differing scales that give the clinician options on reporting clients' functioning in relation to specific activities (e.g., occupational, social, psychological). Another suggestion is to add scales where the clinician could state the adequacy of the client's resources. On Axis I and II, the focus seems to be on giving the clinician more options in diagnosing the severity of the disorder than are offered in the DSM-III-R.

There is a movement towards reorganizing diagnoses from one category to another to allow the clinician to make a quicker and more reliable differential diagnosis (for example, by removing the Schizotypal Personality Disorder from the personality disorder section and placing it under the general heading of Schizophrenia). For those of you who are interested in looking at the research that has gone into these options, the APA will publish its field trials and data analyses in a book entitled *DSM-IV Source Book*.

You need to become familiar with the process by which diagnoses and diagnostic nomenclature are formulated, because your diagnosis of a client can affect whether insurance companies and other providers will pay for your services and for how long.

The Politics of Payment

With the proliferation of PPOs, HMOs, and managed care systems that we now face, accurate and specific diagnoses of clients is necessary. We are all waiting for a much-needed overhaul of the healthcare system in the United States. President Clinton has named this reorganization a number one priority.

Did you know that one of the proposals being presented to the new administration in effect proposes that a national health insurance system would pay only for diagnoses considered "severe"? One of the definitions of "severe" that is being considered is a diagnosis whose etiology can be noted on Axis III (Medical Conditions). Another suggested interpretation of the definition of a "severe" diagnosis is any condition or disorder that would require medication or hospitalization.

The implications of this politicizing of the diagnostics of mental disorders are frightening. Preventative mental health, adjustment disorders, nonmedical stress disorders, anxiety disorders and mood disorders that do not require medication or hospitalization may not be reimbursable. As an example, some clinicians estimate that between 50% and 70% of the U.S. population is dysthymic. Will dysthymia to be considered a "severe" mental condition? If the above criteria of severity are adopted by our political leaders, the vast majority of clients seeking help will not be covered for the most common disorders presented to clinicians on an outpatient basis in a private practice.

The trend in the United States for treating mental disorders is to allow for a maximum of 20 visits per year using a behavioral/cognitive model or a medical model as the primary treatment modality. As clinicians, we have been walked "down the garden path" to a behavioral 5/readjustment paradigm of mental health. The object of treatment is rapidly eroding to include disorders and treatment modalities aimed at keeping a citizen functional, whether or not that individual suffers from a diagnosis that is not amenable to a cognitive/behavioral protocol. Functioning is only one measure of a person's mental health. If clinicians do not stay alert to this political and economic influence on diagnoses and treatment, we will find ourselves acting as agents of governmental policies to keep individuals adjusted to situations (work, school, family settings, etc.) that serve as a collective and unconscious political and corporate system.

Our passive acceptance (and thus acquiescence) of the diagnostic and statistical manuals of the past has been one of the primary ways in which clinicians, for the purposes of receiving immediate reimbursement for treatment, have "worked themselves out of a profession" and thus colluded with the system.

With the coming of national health insurance, expect unnecessary regulations placed within the healthcare system—ostensibly to guard against fraudulent practitioners and unnecessary treatment. More likely, they will dictate that good cases (meaning malevolent and greedy practitioners) will regulate the practice of psychotherapy more than hard-working and honest clinicians.

Clients undergoing psychotherapy, and those who have had psychotherapy in the past, reduce their use of medical care by up to 90%. I do not think the American Medical Association or the insurance companies really want to know whether this estimate is accurate or not. There is too much money involved in denying this type of research. Illness (medical or psychological) is big business.

The underlying concern of therapists should be to continually examine whether we are part of the disease or part of the treatment.

Epilogue: The Spiral Staircase

In your internship and in your practice you will have experienced the "therapeutic honeymoon." This is where, in the early phases of therapy, you are like a knight in shining armor (rescuer) who helps the damsel in distress (client) acquire insight and gain hope. Your client makes rapid and significant progress; improvement seems almost effortless. However, within the first six months, instead of knight and damsel riding off into the sunset, the romantic illusion fades. Reality returns. Clients begin to make telling statements such as "I thought we were getting someplace. Now, I feel like I'm back where we started."

Often, at this point, therapists either implicitly agree or become defensive and disagree with their client's perceptions. I have done both, and to me neither approach felt productive. So, I'd like to offer a way to reframe our understanding of this recurring event.

Most of us tend to think about life as a linear succession of events that starts at some 0-mile marker and stretches forward to our death. As we move through life, we cross over markers that denote significant events and experiences that affected and perhaps changed us. And so it goes, ever forward.

Borrowing from the Irish poet, Yeats, I have begun to conceive of life as a spiral staircase rather than a linear plane. Near the bottom rungs of the staircase (equivalent to our early psychological development) we have the deep childhood experiences that mold and define us. If we are psychologically wounded, betrayed, or abused, then as we ascend that metaphorical staircase, we *will* pass over those sufferings again and again—but each time at a higher level. In other words, we may never fully be free of our early childhood trauma, but we have the opportunity through distance and new insight to form a new, possibly liberating, relationship to it.

As we climb the staircase, we experience movement and differences in depth perception. In therapy, and in life, it is extremely important that your clients understand this concept. They need to see that we do not simply do or feel the same things twice, so long as there has been time or movement (negative or positive) between similar events.

114

Psychotherapy is the process by which we help our clients gain enough insight to see the similarities and differences of how they presently respond to reminders from the past. Does my client who is standing on the thirty-third step of the staircase experience the reprimand of his or her employer the same way he or she felt when, on the third step of the staircase, his or her grammar school principal chided him? He or she may respond affirmatively: "Having my boss say that to me was like having my father yell at me." My response to that is, "I understand that you had similar feelings about seemingly similar events. Do you experience your boss as having total control over your life as your father did when you were three years old? If you do perceive them as the same, are they in fact the same?" How we feel is a matter of an interpretation of an experience, not necessarily the reality of the experience.

Once clients understand this idea, they may lose the unrealistic expectation that life ever becomes completely problem-free, and they are empowered to see more clearly the progress that they make and the benefit that they gain in psychotherapy.

The same insight has helped me in my work as a psychotherapist. At times, when my caseload is down or I have made a mistake that has cost me a relationship with a client, it feels as if my practice and I have failed. I am sorry to report to you that even after 25 years of private practice, I still walk on certain steps of the spiral staircase that are just above the early steps inspiring fear of loss; as a result, they reflect back on my basic insecurities.

No matter how successful we are or will become, we will each pass over the same steps now and again. Hopefully, like our clients, we will be able to perceive the difference in depth between those early steps and where we now stand.

Appendix A

Advertising:
A Legal and Ethical Perspective
by Richard S. Leslie, Legal Counsel

Advertising is an important part of doing business as a healthcare provider. Similarly it plays an important role in the general business world. Healthcare providers, both individual and institutional (hospitals, residential treatment centers, etc.), seem to be advertising much more today than in years past. This is due to a variety of factors but is primarily attributable to the intense competition that exists in the healthcare marketplace for clients and patients, and to the lifting of restrictions on advertising that previously existed. While advertising is now generally considered to be professionally acceptable, there are considerations that practitioners must be aware of to avoid violating the law. This section will address the subject as it pertains to marriage, family, and child counselors and those aspiring to the license.

In the early years of the profession, ethical standards prohibited many forms of advertising. Members were expelled from the association for such violations as bold-face type or box ads in yellow-page advertising. This attitude about "professionalism" was common at that time. Lawyers, for instance, were severely restricted in terms of price advertising, and local bar associations actually prohibited lawyers from charging or advertising fees below the standards set by the association.

As in many other areas of law and public policy, attitudes began to change. The United States Supreme Court, in a case involving lawyer advertising and pricing, clearly established the right for professionals to advertise and to set their own fees. Advertising began to be seen as something that was good for the consumer in that it promoted competition. Today, the right to advertise is clearly established, and many of the prior restrictions have been removed.

It is important for practitioners to understand that advertising can take many forms. Far too many therapists limit their thinking to yellow-page directories. A wide array of newspapers and magazines (both of a general and specific nature) is available. Radio and television advertising are increasingly used by a variety of healthcare providers, as are pamphlets, brochures, announcements, and direct mail. Therapists, like other business people, can use the services of public relations or marketing and advertising consultants who can help to establish a marketing or advertising plan, develop a logo for one's business, and offer a variety of suggestions and services regarding business cards, business name, stationery, and other details pertaining to one's professional image. Consultants can help therapists to promote themselves in line with their competencies and preferences for a particular client population. Care must be taken, of course, when selecting an advertising or marketing consultant, as the unwary or unsophisticated therapist could spend a lot of money with very little result.

The General Rule

Several sections of California law make clear that it is unlawful to advertise in a manner that is false, misleading, or deceptive. False, misleading, or deceptive advertising can be prosecuted as a criminal offense (usually as a misdemeanor, punishable by a fine and/or jail) and can be the basis of a license suspension or revocation proceeding brought by the Board of Behavioral Science Examiners (BBSE). Section 651 of the Business and Professions Code (B & P Code), for instance, states that it is unlawful for any person licensed under Division 2 of the Business and Professions Code (i.e., MFCCs, LCSWs, psychologists, psychiatrists, and other healthcare providers) "to disseminate or cause to be disseminated, any form of public communication containing a false, fraudulent, misleading, or deceptive statement of claim, for the purpose of or likely to induce, directly or indirectly, the rendering of professional services or furnishing of products in connection with the professional practice for which he is licensed. A 'public communication' as used in this section includes, but is not limited to, communication by means of television, radio, motion picture, newspaper, book or list or directory of healing arts practitioners."

The section then explains that a false, fraudulent, misleading, or deceptive statement or claim includes a statement or claim that does any of the following:

1. Contains a misrepresentation of fact

2. Is likely to mislead or deceive because of a failure to disclose material facts

3. Is intended or is likely to create false or unjustified expectations of favorable results

4. Relates to fees, other than a standard consultation fee or a range of fees for specific types of services, without fully and specifically disclosing all variables and other material factors

5. Contains other representations or implications that, in reasonable probability, will cause an ordinarily prudent person to misunderstand or be deceived

Included in the sections of law prohibiting false, fraudulent, misleading, or deceptive advertising for all healthcare practitioners are references to professional business cards, professional announcements, office signs, letterhead, telephone directory listings, and other similar professional notices or devices. The MFCC licensing law, in Section 4980.03(d) of the Business and Professions Code, defines the word *advertise* as follows:

> Advertise, as used in this chapter, includes, but is not limited to, the issuance of any card, sign, or device to any person, or the causing, permitting, or allowing of any sign or marking on, or in, any building or structure, or in any newspaper or magazine or in any directory, or any printed matter whatsoever, with or without any limiting qualification. It also includes business solicitations communicated by radio or television broadcasting.

In another section of the MFCC licensing law dealing with unprofessional conduct, Section 4982(f) of the Business and Professions Code allows the board to revoke or suspend a license or registration (or refuse to issue a license or registration) if a person makes a misrepresentation as to the type or status of a license or registration held, or otherwise misrepresents or permits misrepresentation of his educational qualifications, professional qualifications, or professional affiliations.

When reading all of these sections together, the spirit and intent of the law should be apparent. The purpose of advertising is to accurately inform the consumer about who you are, the type of license you hold, the services you provide, and a host of other information intended to inform and not to mislead, deceive, or misrepresent.

Advertising Specific Information

No exhaustive list of specific items that can or should be advertised exists. These decisions are usually made by the individual practitioner on a case-by-case basis. Section 651 of the Business and Professions Code, however, does contain a list of items that licentiates may advertise, but the section also states that licentiates may advertise "any other item of factual information that is not false, fraudulent, misleading, or likely to deceive." Among the listed items of permissible advertising are:

a. A statement of the name of the practitioner

b. A statement of addresses and phone numbers of the offices maintained by the practitioner

c. A statement of the office hours regularly maintained by the practitioner

d. A statement of languages, other than English, fluently spoken by the practitioner or a person in the practitioner's office

e. A statement that the practitioner is certified by a private or public board or agency, or a statement that the practitioner limits his or her practice to specific fields

f. A statement that the practitioner provides services under a specified private or public insurance plan or healthcare plan

g. A statement of names of schools and postgraduate clinical training programs from which the practitioner has graduated, together with degrees received

h. A statement of publications authored by the practitioner

i. A statement of teaching positions currently or formerly held by the practitioner, together with pertinent dates

j. A statement of the practitioner's affiliations with hospitals or clinics

k. A statement of the charges or fees for services or commodities offered by the practitioner

l. A statement that the practitioner regularly accepts installment payments of fees

m. otherwise lawful images of a practitioner, his or her physical facilities, or of a commodity to be advertised

n. A statement or statements providing public health information encouraging preventative or corrective care

With respect to items k, l, and m, a few comments are in order. Insofar as fees are concerned, the MFCC licensing law does require that MFCCs disclose to their clients or prospective clients, prior to the commencement of treatment, the fee to be charged for professional services, or upon what basis the fee will be computed. It is my belief that acceptance of installment payments should be avoided when possible, since it can lead to fee disputes when the balance owed begins to interfere with the therapeutic relationship. Payment for sessions at the time therapy is performed is usually preferred, but may not always be possible. Any policy regarding installment payments should be clearly presented, preferably in writing.

With respect to commodities, this is generally not applicable to therapists, but I am aware of situations in which therapists have sold products to clients, such as tapes and books. It is my belief, generally, that therapists should not be in the business of selling products to clients, but should have the client purchase or obtain recommended books, tapes, and so on elsewhere. This practice will prevent the client from believing that the therapist is making the recommendation because of the promise of financial reward to the therapist.

Use of License Number in Advertising

While former regulations required the use of the license number in all advertisements, such is no longer the case. Section 1811 of the regulations (Title 16, Chapter 18 of the California Code of Regulations) gives MFCCs an option: either use the exact title of your license in the advertisement (licensed marriage, family, and child counselor is the exact title) and you don't have to use your license number in the ad, or use something other than the exact title (any deviation from the above-described title) and you must use your license number.

Some practitioners do not like to use the license number since it makes them feel like a contractor and, arguably, adds nothing important vis-a-vis consumer protection. Those practitioners can avoid use of the license number by clearly stating the full title of their license. Others who wish to use something other than their full license title, such as marriage and family therapist, or individual and group counseling, must use the license number in the advertisement

Psychotherapist/Psychotherapy

Historically, the use of the above-referenced words in advertising has been a source of some debate. In 1975 an opinion of the California Attorney General's Office cautioned against the use of similar words that could mislead the public into thinking that the practitioner possessed a license that was broader in scope than the MFCC license. Thus, a licensed MFCC who advertises as a psychotherapist, with no further information, and who has a Ph.D. degree following his or her name, might be believed by a consumer to be a psychologist. On the other hand, an examination of several state laws clearly indicates that marriage, family, and child counselors are psychotherapists, do practice psychotherapy, and may advertise such facts.

The solution for those who desire to advertise using such words is to state the exact title of the license in the advertisement. This accomplishes two purposes: it appropriately explains to the consumer what kind of licensee is performing the service, and it allows the practitioner to forego using the license number in the advertisement. While this issue was sometimes heavily debated in the late 1970s and early 1980s, it no longer appears to be a major issue, unless the advertising, when taken as a whole, is misleading or deceptive.

Use of Fictitious Business Name

As a result of the passage of AB 4617 (1988) (the CAMFT-sponsored bill that became law on January 1, 1989), MFCC professional corporations were granted the right to use a fictitious business name. Previously, only sole proprietorships, partnerships, or loose associations were permitted to use fictitious business names. CAMFT sponsored the bill because there was no good reason why those who chose to conduct business in the corporate form should be at a competitive disadvantage.

AB 4617 specified that any person conducting a practice as a marriage, family, and child counselor, whether incorporated or unincorporated, may not use a name that is false, misleading, or deceptive. Thus,

MFCCs who use fictitious business names should take care not to use words or phrases that might lead a reasonable person to believe that they practice under a different license than they possess. Words like *medical, psychological,* and *psychology* should be avoided. Additionally, the name used should not lead the reasonable consumer to believe that MFCCs may diagnose or treat physical conditions.

Certain disclosures are required by licensed marriage, family, and child counselors who conduct their businesses or hold themselves out by use of a fictitious business name (Doing Business As or D/B/A). These disclosures are required whether the practices are incorporated or unincorporated. Disclosures are not required for MFCC corporations that conduct business under their approved corporate names (as registered with the BBSE) or for those individuals who conduct business under their true names.

The specific disclosures required depend on whether the practice is incorporated or unincorporated. If the practice is a marriage, family, and child counseling corporation, the law requires that the client be informed, prior to commencement of treatment, that the practice is conducted by a marriage, family, and child counseling corporation. If the practice is unincorporated, then the client must be informed, prior to the commencement of treatment, of the name and license designation of the owner or owners of the practice.

The law does not specify whether the required disclosures are to be in writing or whether they may be given orally. Thus, either method is permissible. If the disclosure is made orally, it would be prudent for the practitioner to contemporaneously record the fact of such disclosures in the client's record. Since the disclosures must be made prior to the commencement of treatment, the recording would typically be done on the intake sheet or at some other place at the beginning of the record or file.

While some therapists have an aversion to being too "legalistic" or defensive in the conduct of their practices, the safe thing to do is to make the disclosures in writing. This could be done in any number of ways. For instance, the disclosures could be made on the form that many therapists give to their clients prior to the commencement of treatment, wherein the therapist sets out the ground rules of his or her practice and informs the client about a variety of issues (e.g., confidentiality, fees, missed appointments, cancellations, child abuse and other reporting requirements, use of special techniques, theoretical orientation).

Some therapists prefer to comply with the disclosure requirement by asking the client to sign an acknowledgement confirming the fact that the disclosures have been made. Others choose to print the disclosure on letterhead, business cards or announcements, billing statements, advertising materials, or other matter. Oral disclosures coupled with notations in the record should ordinarily evidence compliance.

Telephone Directory Listings/Psychologist

As indicated earlier, yellow pages and other directory listings are considered advertising and all of the rules and restrictions apply. Licensed marriage, family, and child counselors, when placing directory advertising, should make sure that the sales representative understands that they are not psychologists and thus should not be listed under that heading. Unfortunately, some marriage, family, and child counselors do appear under that heading. While some of those listings may not result in disciplinary action (e.g., where the MFCC can prove that he or she did not place the ad, or where the MFCC also holds a license as a psychologist), others may.

MFCCs point out that some psychologists list themselves under the heading "marriage, family, and child counselors" and rely upon that fact to justify their actions. In my opinion, neither listing is appropriate and both may result in licensing board action against the practitioner. Inappropriate yellow-page advertising by MFCCs has led the California State Psychological Association to sponsor AB 3215, a bill that would allow any ten psychologists, under specified circumstances, to sue any person who was, in their opinion, violating the Psychology Licensing Act.

Intern Advertising

Many questions arise when the topic of intern advertising is raised. The regulations do contain some guidance regarding required disclosures, but those regulations do not adequately address the more basic issues. Most interns run into trouble when the advertisement appears to be a promotion of their own practice or business. Generally, such ads do not adequately disclose that the intern is employed by a licensee or other entity, nor do they adequately indicate that the intern works under supervision. It must be remembered that interns can have no ownership or proprietary interest in the business and must be hired as an employee. Additionally, employees usually don't determine the manner, style, or contents of an ad—the employer does.

Interns should take care to check with their employer before committing to any form of advertisement, including business cards. Section 1811 of the regulations states that an unlicensed MFCC Registered Intern may advertise if such advertisement complies with Section 4980.44(e) of the Business and Professions Code by making the required disclosures (inform each client or patient prior to performing any professional services that he or she is unlicensed and under the supervision of a licensed MFCC, LCSW, licensed psychologist, or a licensed physician certified in psychiatry).

Thus, the advertisement must clearly indicate, when read in its entirety, that the intern is not licensed and is not practicing independently. Inclusion of the intern registration number would seem to be required if the registered intern did not identify himself or herself by using the exact title of the registration, but the regulation is somewhat ambiguous in this regard. An intern would be wise, however, to identify himself or herself as an MFCC Registered Intern, and to disclose the name and exact license title of his or her employer or supervisor.

The BBSE has recently revised its guidelines on advertising. Those guidelines are available from the BBSE upon request, and they contain examples for both licensees and interns.

CAMFT's *Ethical Standards for Marriage and Family Therapists* (Part I), contains a section on advertising. Much of the Code can be seen as a restatement of the laws and regulations discussed above, and it contains other useful information and guidelines. It is reprinted here for your convenience.

7. Advertising

Marriage and family therapists engage in appropriate informational activities, including those that enable laypersons to choose marriage and family services on an informed basis.

7.1 Marriage and family therapists accurately represent their competence, education, training, and experience relevant to their practice of marriage and family therapy.

7.2 Marriage and family therapists assure that advertisements and publications, whether in directories, announcement cards, newspapers, or on radio or television, are formulated to convey information that is necessary for the public to make an appropriate selection. Information could include:

1. name, address, telephone number, hours, fee structure, and languages spoken

2. appropriate degrees, state licensure (license number may be required), and CAMFT membership (see 7.8)
3. description of practice

7.3 Marriage and family therapists do not use a name which could mislead the public concerning the identity, responsibility, source, and status of those practicing under that name and do not hold themselves out as being partners or associates of a firm if they are not.

7.4 Marriage and family therapists do not use any professional identification (such as a professional card, office sign, letterhead, or telephone or association directory listing) if it includes a statement or claim that is false, fraudulent, misleading, or deceptive if it a) contains a material misrepresentation of fact; b) fails to state any material fact necessary to make the statement, in light of all circumstances, not misleading; or c) is intended to or is likely to create an unjustified expectation.

7.5 Marriage and family therapists correct, wherever possible, false, misleading, or inaccurate information and representations made by others concerning the marriage and family therapist's qualifications, services, or products.

7.6 Marriage and family therapists make certain that the qualifications of persons in their employ are represented in a manner that is not false, misleading, or deceptive.

7.7 Marriage and family therapists may represent themselves as specializing within a limited area of marriage and family therapy, but may not hold themselves out as specialists without being able to provide evidence of training, education, and supervised experience in settings which meet recognized professional standards.

7.8 Marriage and family therapist clinical, associate, and student members may identify their membership in CAMFT in public information or advertising materials, but they must clearly and accurately represent whether they are clinical, associate, or student members.

7.9 Marriage and family therapists may not use the initials CAMFT following their name in the manner of an academic degree.

7.10 Marriage and family therapists may use the CAMFT logo only after receiving permission in writing from the Association. Permission will be granted by the Association to CAMFT members in good standing in accordance with Association policy on use of CAMFT logo. The association (which is sole owner of its name, logo, and the abbreviated initials CAMFT) may grant permission to CAMFT committees and chartered chapters in good standing, operating as such, to use the CAMFT logo. Such permission will be granted in accordance with Association policy on use of CAMFT logo.

7.11 Marriage and family therapists use their membership in CAMFT only in connection with their clinical and professional activities.

Appendix B

Selling Your Practice:
Ten Provocative Questions

Sherri Ferris, M.S.

What Type of MFCC Business Is Most Salable?

When I moved to the San Francisco Bay Area from Orange County, I mentioned that I had sold my psychotherapy business to a colleague who responded with amazement, stating, "Sherri, don't call what you did a 'business' up here. It will offend the purists." I promptly decided to take a risk in offending my colleagues so that I could explain how, as a therapist, you can have the best of both worlds: be a dedicated, caring clinician and still make money ethically and legally.

Those of you who are entrepreneurial and can develop a heterogeneous group practice featuring multispecialties, men and women, varied mental health licenses, varying ages and orientations, with a diverse physician-referral base, will have more appeal to a buyer than a sole proprietorship with limited referral networks. If you are the only income-producing entity and you leave, why would your patients stay? The argument exists that your patients have a highly personal relationship with you, and, of course, that patients always have the freedom of choice. The patients are not for sale; what is for sale is a functioning business with continuing income generated by independent contractors and good dependable referral sources.

How Can I Place a Value on My Practice?

There must be, based upon a track record, a reasonable expectation that business will continue to grow under proper management. A purchase price can be determined by placing a value on the tangible assets, such as furnishings, and intangible assets, such as goodwill. The IRS and your accountant may determine how the purchase price is allocated to various assets in order to maximize depreciation and improve tax advantages. The following are examples of assets that can be valued to determine the worth of a mental health practice:

- A building and land owned by the seller, which may be sold or retained and leased to the new owner. If rented, the lease would be assigned.

- Patient files and records.

- Fixed assets, such as furniture, equipment, and supplies.

- Intangible assets, such as goodwill, public appeal, and the owner's reputation.

- A Covenant Not to Compete, within a specific distance and time period. Typically the buyer wants to ensure that the seller does not take the proceeds from the sale and start a competing business nearby.

- Contracts with Health Maintenance Organizations or Preferred Provider Organizations and hospital affiliations that may be transferable. These may be intangible, but are useful in determining future referrals.

- Accounts receivable, which may be kept and collected by the seller, who may pay a percentage for their collection by an agency or individual, or may be sold at a discounted rate to the buyer, depending on their aged value. Their value is negotiable. There are advantages and disadvantages to both buyer and seller whether the choice is to keep or sell.

What Is an MFCC Business Worth?

The value of a MFFC business is typically determined by the average of the last four years' gross and net earnings, or occasionally by only the previous fiscal year's gross and net earnings. No business is worth its best year. A typical selling price is one to two years' net or gross earnings, but the price is highly negotiable.

What Are Typical Payment Arrangements?

Businesses may be purchased for a flat fee, which is sometimes a discounted rate to the buyer since he or she carries the risk of success or failure, or by a factor based on the number of ongoing patients. This is typically assessed for not more than four or five years, since there are too many variables in determining the business' productivity for a longer period of time.

The sale agreement can include a minimum and maximum guarantee to protect the buyer and seller, with an option for the seller to reclaim the business if the gross receipts decline below an agreed-upon amount. In the case of a marked increase in success, the buyer can be protected from paying an exorbitant amount to the seller. Much depends on the buyer's ready cash and projected ability to continue a successful business.

To Whom Should I Sell My Practice?

A "clone" with significant financial assets is perhaps the best answer to the question of to whom you should sell your practice. I can't sufficiently emphasize the importance of careful selection to find a buyer who will "carry on the tradition." This means someone who is ethical, who has a keen ability to bond with referral sources and patients, who isn't afraid of working long hours, who has had experience in operating a business, and who is competent at marketing and public relations. Choosing someone of the same sex who has similar therapeutic skills and values will be helpful to your patients.

Optimally, a good choice is someone who has been an associate in your business, and who has familiarity with your patients, referral sources, and office procedures. She or he should be the clinical guru, "the sizzle" who can continue to nurture the referral sources and build new ones, dividing time proportionately between seeing patients, marketing, and business management.

The purchaser cannot be an absentee landlord. If you have a successful business, interested buyers will come to you once you get the word out. It's surprising how fast such news travels. Otherwise, you can advertise in professional association publications or hire a practice sales company who will evaluate your business and find a buyer for you for a fairly substantial percentage.

What Terms Are Contained in an Agreement?

The first step in writing an agreement is to hold initial discussions. (Corporations must document in their corporate minutes the intent to sell.) Prospective buyers are interviewed and, if both parties are sincerely interested, accounting records are shared. These typically include the general ledger, financial statements, bank reconciliations, and records of accounts receivable. Have each sincerely interested party sign an agreement to keep confidential all information, and should business negotiations be terminated, to return all information to you.

The next step is to establish a date of sale and to negotiate terms. A letter of intent delineating both buyer's and seller's positions should be prepared. From this stage forward there will be endless negotiations and revisions. The rule of thumb is "keep it simple." The attorneys will make it complicated enough.

Each party should involve an attorney, to represent his or her best interests, and an accountant, to prepare the forms and documents required by the IRS and to consider the tax consequences involved in such an agreement.

Because of the Bulk Sales Act, a 30-day, interest-bearing escrow account should be opened in both the buyer's and seller's names to ensure that there are no outstanding debts incurred by the seller that would become the responsibility of the buyer. It's often advisable to ask the buyer to deposit the equivalent of three months' operating capital in an account to ensure that there are sufficient funds to cover the overhead during the transition.

What Factors Make the Transfer of Ownership Easier?

Arrange to make the lease assignable (if you have one). Help the new owner to transfer the D/B/A (Doing Business As or fictitious business name). Start initial negotiations with potential buyers at least one year in advance of the date of sale, because it will take twice as long to complete this transaction as you expect. Also, there are always surprises, as when the person who committed to the purchase changes his or her mind. Many calamities are bound to occur, so gather your resiliency.

It is appropriate for the seller to act as a business consultant to the new owner for a specified length of time to ease the transition. It is helpful to provide the buyer with important data, such as lists of referral sources, furniture, equipment, supplies, taxes, licenses and insurance policies, and a list of contracted services, so that the buyer is prepared to pay for or discontinue such services on the renewal date.

If the seller keeps the accounts receivable, he or she should send a letter to all patients with open balances advising them of the billing changes. Letters should be sent to all referral sources and professional colleagues endorsing the new owner and stating the dates of scheduled meetings to facilitate appropriate contacts. Encourage office staff to remain with the new owner, and offer reassurance as needed. Discuss salaries, raises, and contracts with existing employees and independent contractors so there are no surprises.

This is not a time to adopt new policies. Don't redecorate. Don't change personnel. Patients will already be sufficiently traumatized with the many other changes. Try to keep the scheduling and the environment the same. The new owner should also wait a few months to introduce his or her individual taste and personality into the business. It is best to create the impression that "everything remains the same."

What About Your Very Important Patients?

Your patients will definitely feel abandoned, angry, sad, confused, and apprehensive about your plans. They will need to process their separation anxiety, grief, and whatever else this major trigger event will be for them. Prepare them early, and tell them all within a two-week time period. Otherwise, some will tell others before you get a chance to, and the latter will be deeply resentful that they didn't hear the news from you.

Stop taking new patients the last few months unless you know you can accomplish what you need to accomplish in a limited period of time. Sit in on sessions with whomever is taking over treatment to process whatever feelings the transition evokes. Give patients a choice of clinicians, or recommend a good match (in or outside your practice) with whomever you think the patient can work most effectively. You always have a responsibility to do whatever is in the patient's best interest. Agree to transfer records to facilitate continuing treatment.

Give patients a written or oral summary of their progress to give them some measure of where they have been and where you think they might like to go. Ask the patients to write good-bye letters to you, if you think it would help them therapeutically. I exchanged tributes, audiotapes, and letters expressing my feelings about the patients I treated, because I would never ask a patient to do anything I wasn't willing to do myself. My motto has always been, "Take your shoes off before walking through someone else's mind."

Reassure patients that they can write or call long after you are gone. Use your departure as a catalyst for patient change. Give it a positive reframe. Use it as a way of helping each person to see that losses are a part of life, universal, unavoidable, inexorable, but necessary because we grow by losing, leaving, and letting go. Your departure can be an example of life as a transformational process. Validate them for their courage, and don't be afraid to cry—they won't be, because hopefully you have encouraged them along the way.

For those clients who haven't been in for awhile, send an announcement offering a closing session or sessions. Many will need to "check in" one last time and would feel angry if you didn't notify them ahead of time.

If you have groups or have provided supervision, these transitions require appropriate planning and closure. A most impactful way to hold a last group session is to pass around a heart and allow each member to express what is in his or her heart regarding the group experience, with each other and with you. The closure of my sexual abuse group of many years was one of the high points of my therapeutic career, rewarding in the sense that I realized I had indeed played an important role in helping others to process a painful past. This brings me to the next important question—you.

What About Your Mental Health?

Since selling your practice evokes dramatic change in your patients (some of mine got remarkably better when they learned they could manage on their own), you probably will feel quite gratified in the end. However, during the process be prepared for major stress. I developed pruritis, stomatitis, vaginitis, pharyngitis, dermatitis, rhinitis, and mastitis (but I never missed a day). Be certain to receive regular massages, beat a pillow, scream in the privacy of your car, and jog enthusiastically in your gym shoes with names of insurance companies written on the soles. You will tremble when you sign the bill of sale. You will have nightmares that it won't go through. You will learn all the ins and outs of fax machines. You will have dinner more frequently with your attorney than your spouse. And you will doubt your sanity many times over—until you have the check in hand.

Where Can I Find Resources?

Unfortunately, very few resources on selling a psychotherapy business exist. Consult with anyone you know who has actually sold a practice. Find a good business law attorney and an accountant who have had experience in selling mental health practices, and expect to pay them a fortune. They are worth it. Plan ahead. If you are just starting out in practice, develop a business that you can be proud of and that others would love to have!

Appendix C
Handouts

In this appendix, I offer a few different handouts that I use in lectures, seminars, and speaking engagements, and outline their audience and the way in which I use them. Use them as springboards for your own handouts that might supplement your speaking engagements or seminars. Their purpose is to provide quick reference or buzz-words and phrases that operate associatively, in a right-brain way, so they may not be self-explanatory outside of the original context.

Books Helpful for Stress

A bibliography is always an easy and effective handout for a course or seminar. Students and other attendees appreciate being able to explore the subject of interest beyond the limits of the lecture time. Bibliographies also demonstrate that you reference and include the thoughts and ideas of other professionals and thinkers in your work and, by extension, keep well-versed and up-to-date in your area of expertise.

Face it, Embrace it, Erase it

Whenever I am asked to give an inspirational speech regarding my personal philosophy and approach to the world, I bring this handout. The motto, "face it, embrace it, erase it," expresses my overall attitude toward problem situations. The phrase is from a handout I found at a Twelve-step program, which psychotherapy has illuminated for me. Depending on the length of the speech, I either cover all the ideas in detail or quickly define each.

A Little Existential Murder

I use this handout in psychopathology lectures when presenting "a work in progress," a new clinical paradigm on which I have been working. "A Little Murder" is the outline for a model of human suffering, and I use it to present the work in progress to the audience. With the ideas outlined in the handout, I am attempting to design a paradigm that demonstrates how people live inappropriately (or as a good existentialist might say, in bad faith). I let the audience know the purpose behind this handout, and often receive wonderful comments and helpful criticism.

A Laundry List on Love and Work

This handout is part of an on-going seminar series on guest relations in the hospitality industry that I present to hotel and casino workers. In the seminars, I work with professionals in the hospitality industry who provide their expertise on vacationing guests. This handout offers ideas on the nature of people and my assumptions as to "where the hotel guests are coming from." The purpose of this handout is to get the audiences thinking about people who work with people in a service industry, and the dynamics of their interactions.

Theories on Love and Work

I use this handout in many different contexts: with helping organizations, psychology students, and management consultations. It gives people a quick reference guide to psychological theories on what makes for happiness and healthy relationships. I often use it as a springboard for teaching psychology to management—I find that more effective than teaching "management psychology."

Concepts of Existentialism

This is a handout for psychology classes. It provides an overview of a philosophical orientation or school of thought and lists buzz-words or phrases that I use in the lecture. The intention is to aid students by emphasizing the main ideas of the lecture both during the lecture and later when they review their notes.

Books Helpful for Stress

The Joy of Meditation. Jack and Cornelia Addington. DeVorss, 1979.

Illusions. Richard Bach. Delacorte, 1977.

Fit or Fat? Covert Bailey. Houghton Mifflin, 1991.

Beyond the Relaxation Response. Herbert Benson. Berkley Publishing, 1985.

Inner Joy. Harold H. Bloomfield and Robert B. Kory. Berkley Publishing, n.d.

Anatomy of an Illness. Norman Cousins. Norton, 1979.

A New Guide to Rational Living. Albert Ellis. Wheman, n.d.

The Power of Affirmations. Jerry Fankhauser. Fankhauser, 1979.

Type A Behavior and Your Heart. Meyer Friedman and Ray H. Rosenman. Knopf, 1974.

Creative Visualization. Shakti Gawain. New World Library, 1978.

Heal Your Body; You Can Heal Your Life. Louise Hay. Hay House, 1988.

Introduction to Yoga. Richard Hittleman. Bantam, 1969.

Love Is Letting Go of Fear. Gerald Jampolsky. Bantam, 1984.

How to Get Control of Your Time and Your Life. Alan Lakein. NAL-Dutton, 1989.

How to Meditate. Lawrence LeShan. Bantam, 1984.

Mind As Healer, Mind As Slayer: A Holistic Approach to Preventing Stress Disorders. K. Pelletier. Peter Smith, 1984.

Wellness Workbook. John Travis and Regina Ryan. Ten Speed Press, 1986.

Love, Medicine & Miracles. Bernie Seigel. Harper & Row, 1986.

Stress Without Distress. Hans Selye. New York: McGraw-Hill, 1956.

Getting Well Again. O. Simonton, S.M. Simonton and J. Creighton. Jeremy P. Tarcher, 1978.

Face It, Embrace It, Erase It

Say "of course"

Affirm reality

Clarify alternatives

Allow freedom

Bear witness

Remember dominance and submissiveness

Do not compromise

Moment of shame as opposed to guilt

Personal myth

Humor defuses shame

Promises are lies

There are no guarantees

Anger bullies reality

Be yourself

Watch for perversion of need (symptom)

Make an ego dystonic symptom into an ego syntonic alternative

Everybody dies

Everything ends

Honor childlikeness

All choices have positive and negative aspects

There are no victims . . . only volunteers

A Little Existential Murder (Death)

Need

Results in   *hurt*   (that cannot be satisfied)

which is expressed in   *anger*

of which we are   *ashamed*

so we feel we must   *apologize*

and by doing this we forget our own   *need*

and so neglect our   *hurt*

and focus on our   *guilt*

but our   *hurt*   always reminds us of   *rejection*

and the   *rejection*   reminds us of our   *abandonment*

and when   *primates*   are   *abandoned*

they   *die*

A Laundry List on Love and Work

1. When we don't get our needs met from one institution, we project those needs onto the next available institution.

2. People initially seek self-worth and esteem from their family.

3. The state of the current family makes it hard to realize one's needs.

4. The current state of the family is not new.

5. Today's family is mainly composed of narcissistically wounded children and adults.

6. Abuse is passed from generation to generation.

7. People do what they learn.

8. People who are wounded compensate in two ways: a passive-dependent form of depression, or an attempt to fulfill grandiose and unrealistic expectations of the self and others.

9. Need for receiving worth passes from the parent to the teacher to the boss, or to the judge to the warden.

10. Work is an inadequate place in which to get love, but it is an appropriate place to express love through labor. "Work is love made visible."

11. Having "stuff" isn't enough.

12. People are intrinsically valuable.

13. Beware the cultural myth, "People are loved for what they do." Think human beings vs. human doings.

14. Love is unconditional, no matter what we do.

15. Most "haves" trade love for achievement.

16. Worth and self-esteem come from being heard and listened to.

17. Employers who genuinely listen to the needs of their employees and respond to them encourage a productive and loving work environment.

18. There are two things any social institution must provide its people: roots and wings.

19. We rarely sue someone we like . . . who cares for us.

Concepts of Existentialism

Existence precedes essence

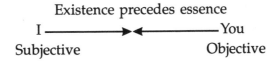

Dominance/Submissiveness Dilemma

Therapeutic Emphasis

Focus		Freedom		
Awareness of choice	=	Responsibility	=	Existential Anxiety

Goals of Therapy	**Communication**	**Assumption**
1. Real reality	What you see is true	People avoid choice to deny freedom
2. Stand uncertainty		
3. Accept absurdity	Affirmation and clarity	
4. Child*like*ness		
5. Recognition of inability to adjust		Personal myth to avoid anxiety and assault
6. Live in good faith (commitment vs. contribution)		

Basic Concepts

1. Nausea (body)
2. Emotions = $\dfrac{\text{announce}}{\text{annihilate}}$
3. Existential anxiety
4. Person in situation
5. Reality is
6. All choices have negative and positive aspects
7. Denial
8. There are no victims
9. Irresponsibility leads to mental illness
10. The engaged encounter
11. All significant relationships are symmetrical
12. All decisions are for the best of all possible reasons
13. All persons are perfect
14. Hell is another person
15. Coefficient of adversity

Death   Responsibility   Freedom   Meaningless   Anxiety   Willingness

Theories of Love and Work

Dysfunctional Family Work Setting

Vertical Relationship

Denies feelings ———— Assumes power

Controller

|

Controllee

Functional Family Work Setting

Horizontal Relationship

Self ———————————— Other

|

Central Relativeness

(Uses feelings to choose behavior)

Maslow's Needs

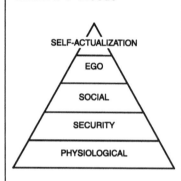

SELF-ACTUALIZATION

EGO

SOCIAL

SECURITY

PHYSIOLOGICAL

Kaiser's Needs
- Security
- Curiosity

Adler's Needs
- Social acceptance
- I am special to someone
- Someone is special to me

Fromm's Love & Freedom
- Freedom "from"
- Freedom "to"
  1. respect
  2. care
  3. know
  4. respond

Jung's Theory of Personality
- Anima (female psyche)
- Animus (male psyche)
- Love and work can be a projection

Toffler's Marriages

First: Romance and child raising
Second: Economic and social growth
Third: Companionship

Elisabeth Kübler-Ross' Stages of Loss
1. Denial
2. Anger
3. Bargaining
4. Depression
5. Acceptance

Causes of Divorce
1. Money, time, work
2. In-laws
3. Having and raising children
4. Social, political, religious points of view
5. Sexuality

> *"Experience is not what happens to you . . . it is how you respond to what happens to you."*
>
> **Aldous Huxley**

Gold's Creative Listening Model
- Recognize differences of male/female orientation
- You can support—you can't help
- Remember you are not alone
- Communicate
- Keep a positive regard
- Complete honesty is destructive
- Have a contract of non-destructiveness
- Acknowledge interdependence
- Make a limited contract:
  a. clear and specific
  b. inclusive and exclusive
  c. open-ended
- Disagreement is OK
  a. recognition
  b. mutual search for alternatives
- Give up historical causes
- Focus on "becoming" (the future)
- Morality is built on full stomachs
- Blame is an avoidance of one's responsibility
- All choices have positive and negative aspects
- There are no victims—only volunteers and/or survivors

Appendix D
Curriculum Vitae

I asked several of my colleagues for copies of their resumes to provide specific examples that might aid you in creating your own resume or curriculum vitae (CV). I have selected an entire resume package sent to me by a clinical and forensic psychologist, Dr. Richard Marsh, who practices in the San Francisco area. Each resume serves a different purpose in Dr. Marsh's practice.

The first resume is a one-page format for clinical and forensic purposes. It presents a quick overview of what Dr. Marsh considers to be the most pertinent information to give to a perspective user of his services, whether it be a client or an agency. Preparing one-page CVs is essential, especially if you interact with the media (newspapers, television, radio). Keep in mind that less is more: people tend to read shorter, concise versions of information you wish to present. The format for this CV is simple and direct. It includes:

1. Professional Credentials

2. Education

3. Experience

4. Personal Information

The second resume is an extension of the one-page format, designed to meet Dr. Marsh's needs for forensic applications. He uses this when he wishes to inform an attorney or an agency of the court of his credentials. The format for this more extensive CV includes:

1. Professional Credentials

2. Education

3. Current Function

4. Case Testimony

Case testimony includes examples of the cases and issues in which he has participated.

The third resume is a four-page format used for both clinical and forensic purposes. It contains the following sections:

1. Objective

2. Professional Credentials

3. Education

4. Experience

5. Current Function

6. Publications

7. Teaching Experience

8. Personal Information

The sections on education and experience are more detailed and extensive than in the shorter formats.

The fourth resume is a five-page format used for presenting Dr. Marsh's specialty in forensic psychology. It includes the following:

1. Objective

2. Professional Credentials

3. Education

4. Current Function

5. Case Testimony

6. Public Presentations and Lectures

7. Publications

8. Teaching Experience

9. Classes and Conferences Attended

10. Personal Information

11. Experience Since Licensure

Each CV focuses on details Dr. Marsh believes would best inform the consumer of his services. Keep the consumers of your services in mind when writing your CV. A CV given to a publisher may require an entirely different format than, say, one prepared for your clients or for public lecturing. Keeping a brief (one page) bio and having an 8 x 10 black and white photo of yourself (preferably with a light background) is most useful when working with the media.

 # I

Richard Charles Marsh, Ph.D.
Clinical & Forensic Psychology
1035 San Pablo Avenue
Suite 7
Albany, California 94706
510-559-8412

CURRICULUM VITAE

PROFESSIONAL CREDENTIALS

Psychologist, State of California, 1976
Marriage, Family & Child Counselor, State of California, 1976
National Register of Health Providers in Psychology, 1978
Superior Court, State of California, County of Alameda
Superior Court, State of California, Contra Costa County
American Psychological Association, 1973
Fellow of the American College of Forensic Psychology
American Psychology—Law Society, APA
Clinical Neuropsychology Division, APA
Child, Youth & Family Services Division, APA
QME: State of California, Dept. of Industrial Relations, Industrial Medical Council
University of California, Berkeley, Extension Division

EDUCATION

Postdoctoral Fellow, UCLA, 1972
Ph.D., Utah State University, 1971

EXPERIENCE

Psychologist: Independent Practice, Beverly Hills (1976–1982), Berkeley & Albany (1983–);
Civil Court work includes assessments re: Child Custody & Visitation and Personal Injury.
Special emphasis in Workers' Compensation and Disability evaluation matters. Criminal
Court work in Los Angeles, Kern, Alameda & Contra Costa County Superior Courts including evaluations of competency to stand trial, NGI, etc.; Dangerousness, W&I; some Juvenile
Court cases. Take referrals from both attorneys for applicants (plaintiffs) and defendants
(carriers) as well as from the Courts and its agencies (PD, DA, Probation, Family Services,
etc.) Current therapy cases of note include work with couples for marital and relationship
problems, injured workers in recovery and return to work context, and children who have
been traumatized by divorce or parental abuse.

PERSONAL INFORMATION

DOB: January, 1942; married; three children, ages 12, 14, and 28 years.

Current: 1/93

#2

Richard Charles Marsh, Ph.D.
Clinical & Forensic Psychology
1035 San Pablo Avenue
Suite 7
Albany, CA 94706
510-559-8412

CURRICULUM VITAE
FOR GENERAL INFORMATION
PROFESSIONAL CREDENTIALS

Psychologist, State of California, 1976
National Register of Health Providers in Psychology, 1978
Fellow of the American College of Forensic Psychology
QME: State of California, Dept. of Industrial Relations, Industrial Medical Council
Expert Witness Lists, Superior Court, State of California, County of Alameda
Expert Witness List, Superior Court, State of California, Contra Costa County
American Psychological Association, 1973
American Psychology—Law Society, APA
Child, Youth, & Family Services Division, APA

EDUCATION

Postdoctoral Fellow, Neurosciences; UCLA, 1972
Ph.D., Psychology; Utah State University, Graduate School,

CURRENT FUNCTION

1983–Continuing. Psychologist in Private Practice, Berkeley & Albany, California; Work weighted in Civil, Workers' Compensation, Child Custody & Criminal Court evaluations and appearances; Also psychological treatment of injured workers and general client population.

CASE TESTIMONY

The following list includes examples of the cases and issues in which I have participated. The list is not exhaustive and most listings represent multiple cases.

Superior Court, Family Division
Contra Costa, Alameda, San Francisco, Ventura, San Diego & Other Counties

Evaluation of Child Custody & Visitation, General Recommendations re: "Best Interests of the Child" and specific issues related thereto such as legitimacy of allegations of sexual abuse and interference with visitation (CC 4700.).

Psychological Evaluation re: Juvenile Offender, Psychopath or Not? (1017/730 Evidence Code)

Duke Case Evaluation re: Adverse Effect on Child of Sale of Family Home (CC 4700.10)

Superior Court, Civil Divisions
Marin, Alameda, San Francisco, Contra Costa & Other Counties

Negligence, Nature & Extent of Psychological Damages in:
Automobile Accident; Automobile Accident with Medical Injury; Wrongful Eviction; Landlord Tenant Dispute; Abuse of Police Powers; Motorcycle Incident; False Imprisonment: Passenger in Aircraft Crash; Pilot in Aircraft Crash; Driver in Truck Crash with fatality; Driver in Automobile Crash with near fatality; Child in Dog Bite Incident; Child in Automobile Crash

Negligence, Nature & Extent of Neuropsychological Damages in:
Head Injury caused by falling debris; Head Injury motorcycle crash

Negligence, Nature of Pre-Injury Psychological Health in a Slip/Fall Accident

Negligence, Malingering

Wrongful Termination, Nature & Extent of Psychological Damages

Superior Court, Criminal Division

Alameda, San Francisco, Kern County

Competency to Stand Trial (Penal Code 1368), Multiple examples

Insane at the Time of the Crime (NGI–Penal Code 1027), Multiple examples

Psychological Evaluation re: PTSD in a Murder Case (Evidence Code 1017/730)

Evaluation of Sexual Offender Status as Pedophile (Penal Code 288.1/1203.03)

Placement of Convicted Felon in Federal Custody (Penal Code 1170.9)

Workers' Compensation Appeals Boards: Alameda, Contra Costa,
San Francisco, Marin, Santa Clara, Los Angeles & Others

Injury to Psyche; AOE/COE; Extent and Duration of Disability; Type and Need for Treatment; Vocation Rehabilitation Eligibility; Apportionment; Fitness for Return to Work

Administrative Law Cases
Alameda, San Francisco, Contra Costa, Marin, Kern, Los Angeles, & Others

EEOC Gender, Sexual Orientation, and Racial Discrimination Evaluations

Determination of Dyslexia eligibility for Bar Exam Privileges

Evaluation of Competency to handle money, decide to marry, choose residence, evaluation of eligibility for state disability

Evaluation of Deferral of Civil Liability re: Mentally Retarded Individual

Evaluation of Dangerousness to Self and Others, Gravely Disabled under W&I 5150; Evaluation of Onset of Mental Disorder following an abandonment of Juvenile by school officials during school sponsored trip

Evaluation of Fitness to Adopt for Adoption Service Agency

#3

Richard Charles Marsh, Ph.D.
Clinical & Forensic Psychology
1035 San Pablo Avenue
Suite 7
Albany, CA 94706
510-559-8412

CURRICULUM VITAE

OBJECTIVE

General Information

PROFESSIONAL CREDENTIALS

Psychologist, State of California, 1976
Marriage, Family & Child Counselor, State of California, 1976
National Register of Health Providers in Psychology, 1978
Fellow of the American College of Forensic Psychology
Expert Witness Lists, Superior Court, State of California, County of Alameda
Expert Witness List, Superior Court, State of California, Contra Costa County
American Psychological Association, 1973
Qualified Medical Examiner, State of California, Dept. of Industrial Relations,
Industrial Medical Council
American Psychology—Law Society, APA
Child, Youth & Family Services Division, APA
Clinical Neuropsychology Division, APA

EDUCATION

Postdoctoral Fellow, Neurosciences, UCLA, Center for Medical Sciences, Brain Research
    Institute & Department of Anatomy, 1972 [in residence: 1971–1972].
Ph.D., Psychology; Utah State University, Graduate School, Department of Psychology,
    . 1971 [in residence: 1969–1971].
M.S., Neuroanatomy & Bioengineering; Purdue University, School of Veterinary
    Medicine, Department of Anatomy, Division of Bioengineering, 1970
    [in residence: 1964–1966].
M.S., Physiology; UCLA, Graduate School, Department of Physiology, 1969
    [in residence: 1968–1969].
A.B., Physiology; University of California, Berkeley, College of Letters & Sciences,
    Department of Physiology, 1964.

EXPERIENCE

1964 Purdue University, Graduate Research Assistant. Worked on anatomy of the Spinal
Column. Taught human physiology to undergraduate students.

1965 Purdue University, Graduate Associate. Worked on and discovered Dendritic bundles, an enabling anatomical condition for ephapsis in the CNS. Taught biology and neuroanatomy to medical and graduate engineering students.

1966 University of Maryland, Medical School Campus, Baltimore; National Institute of Mental Health (NIMH) Predoctoral Fellow. United States Public Health (USPH) Predoctoral Fellow. Worked on biophysical properties of neuronal membranes, Structure activity relationships in the channels for Na+ and K+ fluxes during the nerve impulse. Taught Biology to advanced high school students.

1967 Marine Biological Laboratory, Woods Hole, Massachusetts; NIMH Predoctoral Fellow. Worked on Giant Squid Axon, Mathematical and Physical-chemical models of nerve membrane function.

1968 University of California, Los Angeles; NIMH Predoctoral Fellow. Further research on dendritic bundles.

1969–1971 Utah State University, Graduate Teaching Assistant, Department of Psychology. Dissertation research on Frontal brain function with Operant behavioral baselines, elucidation of pain pathway. Taught physiological psychology, sensory processes, operant conditioning and experimental psychology to undergraduate and graduate students.

1971 University of California, Los Angeles; Brain Research Institute; Postdoctoral Fellow, NIMH, USPH, and Researcher in Neuroscience. Worked on the genesis of the EEG, dendritic bundles, learning in midbrain preparation (cats), and cellular and subcellular mechanisms of learning. Lectured on Neurosciences to medical students.

1972–1974 Eastern Kentucky University, Assistant Professor of Psychology, research and teaching. Development of operant baselines for physiological manipulations. Elucidation of central nervous system mechanisms of operant and respondent conditioning. Taught physiological, experimental, and operant and respondent conditioning to undergraduate and graduate psychology students. Supervised graduate degree programs.

1972–1973 Kentucky State Mental Hospital, Lexington; Ward Intern. Schizophrenia and alcoholic inpatient treatment and diagnoses.

1974–1976 Los Angeles County Mental Health Service Staff Psychologist and Intern. Full-range exposure to outpatient treatment modalities in community mental health setting. Assessment with interview and objective and projective psychological testing; psychodiagnostics; individual & group psychotherapy; staffings with multidisciplinary team; forensic reports and appearances; disability determinations.

1974–1976 Psychological Assistant to Private Practitioner (Wm. Zehv, Ph.D.). Worked with physicians, Beverly Hills and San Fernando Valley. Evaluations and treatment of orthopedic medical cases for Workers' Compensation and private surgical patients. Taught at Los Angeles Valley College, General, Child, Advanced Child, and Abnormal Psychology to undergraduate students.

1976–1982 Private Practice Psychologist, Beverly Hills, California. Practice heavily weighted with medical consultation and Workers' Compensation issues. Individual and group psychotherapy; psychodiagnostics; forensics; All age clients. Symposia given on Medical Patient Personality, Psychodiagnoses, and Adult Development.

1979–1980 Medper Corporation, Project Team Director, Medper Project. Developed a special analysis of the Minnesota Multiphasic Personality Inventory (MMPI) for medical patients. Field validation and standardization.

1977–1979 Consultant Psychologist, San Fernando Valley Problem Back Pain Clinic. Interdisciplinary staffings with medical specialists [orthopedic surgeons, radiologists, neurosurgeons, rheumatologists, general practitioner].

1981–1982 Director, R.C. Marsh, Ph.D. & Associates. Diagnostic and therapeutic work with inpatient brain and spinal cord impaired population; training and administration of subordinate psychologists and facility staff.

1981–1985. Chief Executive Officer, Medper Corporation. Directed the activities of a diagnostic testing service resulting from the Medper Project.

1983 Certified Masters and Doctoral professionals in Clinical Hypnotherapy under the auspices of Board of Behavioral Science Examiners, State of California. Certification included training and clinical supervision.

1983 Center for Neuro Skills, Chairman, Department of Psychology. Psychological Assessment and treatment of head trauma cases; administration of department in a rehabilitation center.

1985–1987. Instructor, University of California, Extension Division. Courses in Somatic Symptom Analysis (How to distinguish Organic vs. Psychological) and Psychodiagnostics (DSM III).

CURRENT FUNCTION

1983—Continuing. Psychologist in Private Practice, Berkeley & Albany, California. Work weighted in Workers' Compensation, Child Custody, Civil & Criminal Court evaluations and appearances, including lecturing; Also psychological treatment of injured workers and general client population. Some Conservatorship & Sexual Offender evaluations.

PUBLICATIONS

Marsh, R.C. *"The Marsh Letter,"* an interdisciplinary newsletter addressing forensic psychological issues shared by psychologists, attorneys, and medical doctors; published bimonthly in Berkeley, California, February, 1986—November, 1988.

Marsh, R.C. Workers' compensation cases in California: New regulations for rating of permanent disability. *American Journal of Forensic Psychology*, Volume 7(2):59–68, 1989.

Marsh, S.E.; Marsh, R.C. & Settle, R.B. MDCMPT: a computer program for the analysis of a short form MMPI. *Medper Inc. Publication Document*. Chatsworth, California, 1981. [Confidential and proprietary]

Marsh, R.C. Medical patient personality inventory, a manual. Medper, Inc. Publication Document. Chatsworth, California, 1981.

Combs, S.M. & Marsh, R.C. Abstract behaviors analyzed in terms of a multiple schedule with positive and negative reinforcement components. American Psychological Association, Montreal, Canada, 1973.

Cyrulnik, R.A.; Anninos, P.A. & Marsh, R.C. Complex symptomatology simulated by unstructured neural nets. *Canadian Journal of Neurological Sciences*, 1974, 1:17–22.

Marsh, R.C. Comparative cytoarchitecture of the spinal cord grey matter in the pig and cat: does Rexed's schema apply to the pig? *Acta Anatomica*, 1972, 83:435–439.

Marsh, R.C. The effects of frontal brain ablation on escape behavior. Ph.D. Dissertation, Utah State University, 1971.

Marsh, R.C.; Matlovsky, L. & Stromberg, M.W. Dendritic bundles exist. *Brain Research*, 1971, 33:273–287.

Marsh, R.C. Cytoarchitecture of the pig spinal cord grey matter and a special study into the interrelationships of dendrites. M.S. Thesis, Purdue University, 1970.

Marsh, R.C. Physiology—the discipline. *Perspectives in Biology and Medicine*, 1969, 12:369–372.

Summary: 4 international scientific journal articles printed and circulating, 2 corporate documents, 2 formal University Theses, several publications and presentations at the state and national level.

TEACHING EXPERIENCE

Summary: 7+ years full-time equivalent. Purdue, UCLA, Utah State University, Eastern Kentucky University, Los Angeles City College, Los Angeles Valley College, University of California Extension. Symposia [private practice]. Highest academic status: Assistant Professor of Psychology.

PERSONAL INFORMATION

DOB: January 20, 1942
married
three children,
ages 12, 14, 28 years
excellent health

Current: 1/93

 # 4

Richard Charles Marsh, Ph.D.
Clinical & Forensic Psychology
1035 San Pablo Avenue
Suite 7
Albany, CA 94706
510-559-8412

CURRICULUM VITAE

OBJECTIVE

General Information

PROFESSIONAL CREDENTIALS

Psychologist, State of California, 1976
Marriage, Family & Child Counselor, State of California, 1976
National Register of Health Providers in Psychology, 1978
Fellow of the American College of Forensic Psychology
Expert Witness Lists, Superior Court, State of California, County of Alameda
Expert Witness List, Superior Court, State of California, Contra Costa County
American Psychological Association, 1973
American Psychology—Law Society, A Division of the APA
APA Division of Child, Youth, & Family Services
Qualified Medical Examiner, State of California, Dept. of Industrial Relations,
Industrial Medical Council
Clinical Neuropsychology Division, APA

EDUCATION

Postdoctoral Fellow, Neurosciences; UCLA, Center for Medical Sciences, Brain Research
    Institute & Department of Anatomy, 1972 [in residence: 1971–1972].
Ph.D., Psychology; Utah State University, Graduate School, Department of Psychology,
    1971 [in residence: 1969–1971].
M.S., Neuroanatomy & Bioengineering; Purdue University, School of Veterinary
    Medicine, Department of Anatomy, Division of Bioengineering, 1970
    [in residence: 1964–1966].
M.S., Physiology; UCLA, Graduate School, Department of Physiology, 1969
    [in residence: 1968–1969].
A.B., Physiology; University of California, Berkeley, College of Letters & Sciences,
    Department of Physiology, 1964.

CURRENT FUNCTION

1983–Continuing. Psychologist in Private Practice, Berkeley & Albany, California; Work
weighted in Civil, Workers' Compensation, Child Custody & Criminal Court evaluations and
appearances; Also Psychological Treatment of Injured Workers and General Client Population.

1985–1987 Instructor, University of California, Extension Division. Courses in Somatic Symptom Analysis (How to distinguish Organic v. Psychological) and Psychodiagnostics (DSM III). In Review for Fall '93: Forensic Psychology.

CASE TESTIMONY

The following list includes examples of the cases and issues in which I have participated. The list is not exhaustive and most listings represent multiple cases.

Superior Court, Family Division
Contra Costa, Alameda, San Francisco, Ventura, San Diego & Other Counties

Evaluation of Child Custody & Visitation, General Recommendations re: "Best Interests of the Child" and specific issues related thereto such as legitimacy of allegations of sexual abuse, interference with visitation, and substantial change in circumstances, (CC 4700.);

Psychological Evaluation re: Juvenile Offender, Psychopath or Not? (1017/730 Evidence Code);

Duke Case Evaluation re: Adverse Effect on Child of Sale of Family Home (CC 4700.10);

Superior Court, Civil Division
Marin, Alameda, San Francisco, Contra Costa, & Other Counties

Negligence, Nature & Extent of Psychological Damages in:
   Automobile Accident associated with Medical Injury;
   Wrongful Eviction;
   Landlord Tenant Dispute;
   Abuse of Police Powers;
   Motorcycle Incident;
   False Imprisonment:
   Slip/Fall of Handicapped Individual with failure to meet requirements for
       handicapped facility by private business;
   Passenger in Aircraft Crash;
   Pilot in Aircraft Crash;
   Driver in Truck Crash with fatality;
   Driver in Automobile Crash with near fatality;
   Child in Dog Bite Incident;
   Child in Automobile Crash;
Negligence, Nature & Extent of Neuropsychological Damages in:
   Head Injury caused by falling debris;
   Head Injury motorcycle crash;
Negligence, Nature & Extent of Learning Disability Damages in an automobile crash;
Negligence, Nature of Pre-Injury Psychological Health in a Slip/Fall Accident;
Malingering in Automobile Accident;
Wrongful Termination, Nature & Extent of Psychological Damages.

Superior Court, Criminal Division
Alameda, San Francisco, Kern County

Competency to Stand Trial (Penal Code 1368), examples: Murder, Possession & Sale of Illicit Drugs, Assault with a Deadly Weapon, Battery with Injury;

Insane at the Time of the Crime (NGI—Penal Code 1027), examples: Murder, Kidnapping, Robbery, Burglary;

Mental Illness as to Premeditation and Deliberation in Murder (Penal Code 187);

Diversion of Mentally Retarded Offender from Criminal Justice System to Mental Health Department, examples: Battery, Burglary;

Psychological Evaluation re: PTSD in a Murder Case (Evidence Code 1017/730);

Evaluation of Sexual Offender Status as Pedophile (Penal Code 288.1/1203.03);

Evaluation of Sexual Abuse of Child

Placement of Convicted Felon in Federal Custody (Penal Code 1170.9);

Workers' Compensation Appeals Boards

Alameda, Contra Costa, San Francisco, Marin,
Santa Clara, Los Angeles, & Others

Injury to Psyche;

AOE/COE;

Extent and Duration of Disability;

Type & Need for Treatment;

Vocation Rehabilitation Eligibility;

Apportionment;

Fitness for Return to Work;

Administrative Law Cases

Alameda, San Francisco, Contra Costa, Marin, Kern, Los Angeles, Others

EEOC Gender, Sexual Orientation, and Racial Discrimination Evaluations;

Determination of Dyslexia Eligibility for Bar Exam Privileges;

Evaluation of Competency to handle money, decide to marry, choose residence;

Evaluation of Eligibility for State Disability;

Evaluation of Deferral of Civil Liability re: Mentally Retarded Individual;

Evaluation of Eligibility for Regional Center Services;

Evaluation of Dangerousness to Self & Others, Gravely Disabled under W&I 5150; Evaluation of Onset of Mental Disorder following an abandonment of Juvenile by school officials during school sponsored trip;

Evaluation of Fitness to Adopt for adoption service agency

PUBLIC PRESENTATIONS AND LECTURES

Numerous symposia and lectures; including presentations to Forensic, Insurance, & Medical groups; service organizations; and radio and television news media. Presentations typically relate to the functions and services of Forensic Psychology, the psychology of being in a litigation, patient compliance, psychodiagnostics, psychological testing, treatment planning, professional relations, the psychology of the medical patient, and the psychological & organic causes of somatic symptoms.

PUBLICATIONS

Marsh, R.C. Workers' compensation cases in California: New regulations for rating of permanent disability. *American Journal of Forensic Psychology*, Volume 7(2):59–68, 1989.

Marsh, R.C. *"The Marsh Letter,"* an interdisciplinary newsletter addressing forensic psychological issues shared by psychologists, attorneys, and medical doctors; published bimonthly in Berkeley, California, February, 1986–November, 1988.

Marsh, S.E.; Marsh, R.C. & Settle, R.B. MDCMPT: a computer program for the analysis of a short form MMPI. Medper Inc. Publication Document. Chatsworth, California, 1981. [Confidential and proprietary]

Marsh, R.C. Medical patient personality inventory, a manual. Medper, Inc. Publication Document. Chatsworth, California, 1981.

Cyrulnik, R.A.; Anninos, P.A. & Marsh, R.C. Complex symptomatology simulated by unstructured neural nets. *Canadian Journal of Neurological Sciences*, 1974, 1:17–22.

Combs, S.M. & Marsh, R.C. Abstract behaviors analyzed in terms of a multiple schedule with positive and negative reinforcement components. American Psychological Association, Montreal, Canada, 1973.

Marsh, R.Ch. Comparative cytoarchitecture of the spinal cord grey matter in the pig and cat: does Rexed's schema apply to the pig? *Acta Anatomica*, 1972, 83:435–439.

Marsh, R.C. The effects of frontal brain ablation on escape behavior. Ph.D. Dissertation, Utah State University, 1971.

Marsh, R.C.; Matlovsky, L. & Stromberg, M.W. Dendritic bundles exist. *Brain Research*, 1971, 33:273–287.

Marsh, R.C. Cytoarchitecture of the pig spinal cord grey matter and a special study into the interrelationships of dendrites. M.S. Thesis, Purdue University, 1970.

Marsh, R.C. Physiology—the discipline. *Perspectives in Biology and Medicine*, 1969, 12:369–372.

TEACHING EXPERIENCE

Summary: 7+ years full-time equivalent: Purdue; Private High School in Baltimore, Maryland; UCLA; Private Elementary & Junior High School in Los Angeles; Utah State University; Eastern Kentucky University; Los Angeles City College; Los Angeles Valley College; & University of California Extension.

Highest academic status: Assistant Professor of Psychology.

CLASSES AND CONFERENCES ATTENDED

Psychometric Evaluation of Brain Injury

Human Sexuality
Sexual Abuse
Hypnosis & Hypnotherapy
Adult Developmental Processes
Cognitive Behavioral Therapy
Psychodiagnostics
MMPI in Forensic Applications

PERSONAL INFORMATION

DOB: January 20, 1942
married; excellent health
three children, ages 12, 14, 28 years

EXPERIENCE SINCE LICENSURE

1976–1982 Private Practice Psychologist, Beverly Hills, California; Practice heavily weighted with Medical Consultation and Workers' Compensation issues. Individual and Group Psychotherapy; Psychodiagnostics; Forensics; All age clients. Symposia given on Medical Patient Personality, Psychodiagnoses, and Adult Development.

1977–1979 Consultant Psychologist, San Fernando Valley Problem Back Pain Clinic; Interdisciplinary staffings with medical specialist [orthopedic surgeons, radiologists, neurosurgeons, rheumatologists, general practitioners].

1979–1980 Medper Corporation, Project Team Director, Medper Project; Developed a special analysis of the Minnesota Multiphasic Personality Inventory (MMPI) for medical patients. Field validation and standardization.

1981–1982 Director, R.C. Marsh, Ph.D. & Associates, Diagnostic and therapeutic work with inpatient brain and spinal cord impaired population; training and administration of subordinate psychologists and facility staff.

1981–1985 Chief Executive Officer, Medper Corporation; Directed the activities of a diagnostic testing service resulting from the Medper Project.

1983 Certified Masters and Doctoral professionals in Clinical Hypnotherapy under the auspices of Board of Behavioral Science Examiners, State of California. Certification included training and clinical supervision.

1983 Center for Neuro Skills, Chairman, Department of Psychology, Psychological Assessment and treatment of head trauma cases; administration of department in a rehabilitation center.

Current: 1/93

Appendix E
Gold's Notes and Cheatsheets

Over the years I have taught both undergraduate and graduate psychology classes. For my classes and seminars that run a day or more, I prepare handout booklets which I call *Gold's Notes.* In each booklet I include a section called Cheatsheets. A Cheatsheet is condensed information on a specific topic. Many former students who are now practicing clinicians have remarked to me how useful these Cheatsheets have been in their private practice, so I offer them to you here.

On the following pages are Cheatsheets that come from the handout booklet called *Gold's Notes on Psychopathology.* I have selected pages from two sections: the first section on goals and interventions; the second on diagnosis and treatment. These Cheatsheets are modified and changed as I become aware of new and appropriate information.

If you teach, conduct seminars, or speak at conferences regularly, you might find it useful to design similar handouts. After a while, you will have developed a set of resource materials that can not only aid you in your practice, but can be given out to professional and lay audiences before whom you speak. Add your name and phone number to the bottom of the handouts so people will know who you are and be able to contact you. The book you have just read is a direct result of notations, quick references, handouts, and Cheatsheets that I have accumulated over the last two decades.

Why not begin *your* book today?

Cheatsheets on Goals and Interventions

These Cheatsheets are very useful for people studying for vignette responses of oral examinations. They are quick reference guides on the goals and interventions of different theoretical orientations.

Working in Family Therapy

Goals

Closeness vs. enmeshment

Good problem solving

Resolution of hierarchies

Cooperation

Open communication

Flexibility

Ability to survive life changes

Spontaneity

Support

Riddance of scapegoat or
　identified patient

Unity

Tolerance of anxiety

Learn how to play

Individuation

Less isolation—extended family
　into community

Sense of family boundaries

Interventions

Sculpting

Mapping

Roleplaying

Geno-Grams

Generational scripts

Tracking

Accommodation

Restructuring:
　systems recomposition
　symptom focusing
　structural modification

Co-therapist—teaming

Family-of-origin work

Paradoxical intervention

Restraining strategies

Prescribing strategies

Positioning

Re-framing

Positive connotation

Joining

Directives

Enactment

Task setting

Family myths

Goal setting

Creating crisis—increasing
　interpersonal stress

Defining of problem

Siding

Exonerating

Reexamining cut-offs

Double-bind

Working with Children

Goals

Normal developmental pattern
End of neurosis/psychosis
Academic achievement
Ability to grieve
Normal affect
Cooperation
Self-esteem
Ego strength
Resolution of separation anxiety
Ability to relate with peers
Appropriate gender identity

Interventions

Verbal techniques:
    three wishes
    what animal are you?
Drawing
Painting
House-tree-person
Testing
Sand table
Storytelling
Play
Games
Family intervention
Multiple-diagnostic sessions
School visits
Parent interviews
Home visits
Consulting colleagues
Toys, tools, things
Humor
Roleplaying
Working alliance with "secret friend or monster"
Interpretation through metaphor (myths and stories)

Working with Behavioral/Cognitive Disorders

Goals

Loss of symptoms
Specific behavioral changes
Objective signs of movement
Happiness (Beck)
Rational decision making (Ellis)
Control of self

Interventions

Assertion training
Aversion training
Successive-approximation techniques
Desensitization
Sensate-focus techniques
Token economy
Reinforcement
Modeling
Guided participation
Symbolic modeling
Restructuring cognitive statements
Conditioning
Behavior rehearsal
Visualization
Covert sensitization
Anchoring behaviors

Working with Psychodynamic Therapy

Goals	Interventions
Insight	Interpretation
Consciousness	Confrontation
Conscious awareness	Clarification
Loosening of symptoms	Working through
Reality principle	Empathy
Ability to relate—love—intimacy	Silence
Autonomy	Talk
Flexibility	Free association
Combination of dependence and independence (interdependence)	Working alliance
	Abreaction—catharsis
	Suggestion
Maturity	Listening
Responsibility	Dream work
Sublimation	Projective tests
Self-assertion	Fantasies
Appropriate affect	Interpreting transference
Control of behavior	Interpreting resistance
Freedom from neurotic defenses	"Going with" resistance
Ability to fail	Analyzing resistance before content
Self-actualization	
Ability to see one's limitations	Ego before id
Acceptance	Beginning with surface
Ego-strength	Active imagination
Self-esteem	Voice dialogue
Motivation	Roleplaying psychodrama
	Body work
	Empty-chair technique
	"I" statements
	Working with ambivalence
	Symbol interpretation—personal/universal
	Visualization
	Unconditional positive regard
	Encounter
	Hypnosis

Working with Elderly and Child Abuse

Goals

Stopping the abusive behavior
Learning other ways to discipline
Learning other ways to deal with frustration, anger, etc.
Raising self-esteem
Forgiveness and acceptance
Nonseparation of geriatrics

Interventions

Instill hope
Information and realistic understanding
Universality of experience
Altruism—giving and receiving support and reassurance
Co-Therapist—mother-father models
Corrective recapitulation of primary family group
Family therapy techniques
Development of social techniques
Incorporating imitative behavior
Interpersonal learning
Insight
Catharsis through abreaction and verbalization
Relationship
Working through of transference
Existential factors—life and death
Responsibility
Consultation, visiting nurses
Self-help groups
Network development
Behavioral techniques for dealing with anger and rage

Cheatsheets on Diagnosis and Treatment

These Cheatsheets, like the Cheatsheets on goals and interventions, are helpful for people studying for vignette responses of oral examinations. They are also useful when filling out mental health treatment reports for managed-care companies.

I have included Cheatsheets for the nine most-used diagnostic categories based on requests from audiences and from consultations with authors regarding psychological material in their fiction and nonfiction. Each Cheatsheet contains the following categories:

Pathology
The specific signs and symptoms

Mood and Affect
The overall pervasive feeling-tone and the specific responses

General Appearance
Physical evaluation of the client

Sensorium/Intellect
The client's orientation in time, place, and person

Patient's Stream of Thought
The clinician's perception of the client's thought, speech, and writing patterns

Treatment
The current accepted forms of treatment

Schizophrenia

Pathology

Hebephrenic—silly
Catatonic—rigid
Paranoid ideation
Thought disorder
Weirdness
Hallucinations
Delusions
The Four A's:
    autism
    affect
    association
    ambivalence
Disorganization
Schizophrenogenic family
    and/or biological history

Mood and Affect

Flat or peculiar affect
Unusual response in terms of
    feelings
Suspicious

General Appearance

Disheveled
Unaware of appearance
Poor hygiene
Sometimes bizarre

Sensorium/Intellect

Autism
Preoccupied with self, little
    awareness of outside
Spotty distortions

Patient's Stream of Thought

Loose association
Ambivalence (love-hate)
Word salad—made up words
Disconnected information
Lots of confusion in terms of
    time, people, logic (therapist's
    normal logic doesn't work)

Treatment

Use psychiatric help, medication
    evaluation
Have to like to work with them
Have a sense of humor
Look for islands of health
Relationship is a tool
Not a lot of uncovering and
    insight
Give structure to life
Give some sense of control
Develop basic primitive trust
Master daily living
Ego building
Lots of encouragement
Advice giving
Therapist's actions speak louder
    than words
Short, direct information—not
    long interpretation
Search for real issues
Feelings—not content
Therapist is reality
Don't argue
Offer alternate possibilities
Work with significant others
Later get into conflict material—
    not to resolve but to get it out
    on the table, so patient can
    monitor self

Organic Mental (Brain) Disorder

Pathology

Acute or chronic
Prenatal
Postnatal
Injuries
Fever
Drugs
Chemicals
Toxicity
Alcohol
Brain Tumors

Mood and Affect

OK but will be embarrassed if
  they can't answer
Some inappropriate affect

General Appearance

Glaring appearance in one area
Gait problems
Balance
Gesticulations—hand gestures
Physical manifestations

Sensorium/Intellect

Gross impairment in many areas
  except for long past memory
  and vocabulary
Spotty deterioration—areas not
  able to track
Loss of recent memory
Loss of concentration
Vocational impact

Patient's Stream of Thought

Slurred speech
Disorganization
Meandering—losing the point
Overt confabulation to cover up
  not knowing

Treatment

Acute; clears up with proper
  medical care
Chronic:
    medical care important
    help make connections
    environment with emphasis on
      protection
Include family and/or social
  support system in treatment
  whenever possible

Depression

Pathology

Sleeping problems
Eating problems
No pleasure
Exogenous or biological base
In general, a defense against introjected hostility
Always restricts interpersonal interaction
Burdened and anxious
Overwhelmed
Impatient to get past complaints

Mood and Affect

Slowed
Dismal—low
Saddened
Fatigue
Lots of expressed neediness and pain
Agitated

General Appearance

Doesn't care
Hopeless
Great deal of apology

Patient's Stream of Thought

Mostly talks about symptoms
Lot of self-accusation
Ancient "shoulds"
Progressive withdrawal
"Nobody cares"
Unexpressed anger initially
Always suicidal risk—assess

Sensorium/Intellect

Confusion that is "I don't care"— too much trouble to sort out
Tired of it
Hypochondriac
Not able to focus because it takes too much energy
Nothing works

Only interested in self, yet wants approval
Judgmental of self
Indecisive

Treatment

Major defenses: introjection and denial
Get into suicidal material directly
Rate suicidal potential (may want second opinion)
Must consider medication
Patient needs to feel can depend on therapist
Reassure
Be available—particularly in relationship
Call in reinforcements in person's support situation (relieves stress on patient and therapist)
Direct approach—authoritative— be good mother
Try to get patient to do something for self
Help self-esteem
Long-range goals aimed at dealing with unexpressed or repressed anger—get in touch with things around which there is anger
Lots of modeling and giving permission
Lots of old guilt—has to do with "Why am I so worthless?"

Suicide

1. Is there a plan?
2. Are there the means (realistically)?
3. Have lots of things happened recently?
4. Is the person alone?
5. Has the person sustained recent losses?
6. Is the person getting affairs in order?

Obsessive/Compulsive Disorder and Obsessive Personality Disorder

Pathology

Dogma to overcome doubt
Hardest to work with—feels put
   down
Unfriendly
Sticky quagmire
Often psychotic stuff underneath
Rigidity to defend
Lot of emotional insecurity, in
   terms of identity figures
Products of irregular emotional
   experience
On continuum with paranoia

Mood and Affect

Good presentation
Rational
Definite and positive (absolute)
Even, tense mood
Black and white
Sounds like a know-it-all
Humorless

General Appearance

Neat and orderly
Punctual
Rude
Ritualistic
Usually a "pigpen" someplace in
   life

Sensorium/Intellect

Opinionated
Intense
Driven
Cranky and crabby
Impatient
Stubborn
Aware of every detail
No hunches
Very dogmatic
Must be right

Patient's Stream of Thought

Ask for manual to live by
Coming because of somebody else
Expect rules
Many fears:
   of humiliation
   being disliked
   being out of step
Subrosa fear about being
   inadequate

Treatment

Consider medication depending
   on degree of disability
Don't get caught in
   intellectualization or arguments
Build self-esteem in terms of
   where the person makes
   emotional investment
Take away doubts
Get person to arrive at some
   inescapable conclusion
Help person explore
   priorities—by questions and
   suggesting alternatives
Breakthrough produces resistance
   and anger
Emphasize agreements on issues
Use a little humor
Help live more comfortably and
   let those around them
   live—take heat off family
Confrontation is not helpful
Often patients have relied on
   fundamental religious systems
Support purposeful superego

Bipolar Disorder (Manic Depression)

Pathology

Find out history
Mood disorder
Hereditary
Biological base
European and Mediterranean descent (Greek, Italian, Jewish, South African)
Correlation with alcoholism

Mood and Affect

Exaltation
Hostility
Depression—down and hopeless

General Appearance

Affect usually correlates with up or down mood
Pressured
Sometimes bizarre

Sensorium/Intellect

Super-aware in manic phase
Depressed—unobserving of everything
Oriented in time and place, but confused
Agitated
Flight of ideas in both phases
Mania feels good

Patient's Stream of Thought

Self-accusation
Self-deprecation
Gets nothing from around them
Never able to love or be loved
Minimal history in early years
Poor judgment
Grandiosity in manic phase
Very unhappy about manic phase
Aware when manic phase comes on
Usually comes on gradually

Treatment

Call in psychiatric help
Families need lots of help
Need protection
Control acting out
Lithium carbonate keeps person stable—often given in manic phase
Keep in treatment
Once-a-year check-ups:
    psychological
    medical
Tendency to stop taking meds in 2nd or 3rd year
Involve family in medication regime

Somatoform Disorder (Psychosomatic)

Pathology

Somatizes conflicting feelings
Cuts across many areas
Association between kind of
   condition that develops and
   kind of personality
Constitutional makeup plays a
   part
Ulcer—unallowed dependency
Colitis—anger
Dermatitis—unexpressed anger
Prevalent secondary gain
Denial

Mood and Affect

Marked anxiety about symptoms
Quality of apprehension

General Appearance

Nothing significant

Sensorium/Intellect

Nothing significant

Patient's Stream of Thought

Preoccupation with illness and
   death
Nobody pays attention to them
Number of doctors involved
Resistance to the fact that it is
   emotional

Treatment

Listen to a lot of rehash
Review medical history and still
   be supportive
After 3 weeks or so, spend less
   time on symptoms
Needs a lot of support
Therapist becomes very
   important
Often finds new symptoms once
   cause-and-effect relationship
   is seen as statement of feelings
Symptom makes "statement" of
   feeling that patient can't
   make
Go with ego strengths—support
   what patient does
Help patient see it is not just
   body that's important
Move person to other areas
Often capable of using insight
Increased passivity and
   dependency
Determine what illness means
Focus on secondary gains

Anxiety Disorder

Pathology

Normal, useful commodity if
   not out of hand
Indicator of internal conflict
Somatoform disorders
Can be raised or lowered by
   therapist
One immediately wants to
   reassure

Mood and Affect

Desparate, panicky quality
Good reality testing
Very conflicted (important)
Feeling helpless
Down and agitated

General Appearance

Nervous
Sweaty
Eats a lot
Blushes
Has hives
Chain smokes

Sensorium/Intellect

Urgent, apprehensive and jumpy
Intact—no distortions
Symptoms are ego-alien
Lot of concern about symptoms
Psychic and physiological
   distress

Patient's Stream of Thought

Preoccupation with panic
Wonder if going crazy
Very sensible
Somewhat disorganized
Hypochondriacal

Treatment

Easiest to treat
Identify conflict
Connection between old conflict
   and current conflict
Something touches off old
   conflicts—need to deal with
   these conflicts
What does person most
   disapprove of in self?
Lot of ventilation and
   clarification
Pace is important—don't move
   too quickly
Lot of support and reassurance
History very important
Not usually a lot of guilt
Support—support—support

Histrionic and Dissociative Disorders

Pathology

Disturbance of sense of reality
Behavior makes unconscious
    statement—fairly specific
Somatoform disorders
Conversion
Amnesia
Déjà vu
Very sympathetic
"So" distressed and "so" nice
Fragile
Needs liking, caring, and
    sympathy
Has demanding significant other
Is envious of friends
Make good patients—high
    incidence of positive
    transference—no oedipal
    resolution

Mood and Affect

Mood swings are noticeable
Labile in affect (changeable)—
    maybe 4 or 5 changes an hour
Lacking in curiosity
Inappropriate affect with content
Unappreciated
Like spoiled child
Pouts
Willful

General Appearance

Overdone in dress and looks
Flamboyant, colorful, like
    budding actor or model
Dramatic, such as heavy makeup
Often female
Flightiness

Sensorium/Intellect

(Self-presentation)
Silly, giggly, giddy
Slightly inappropriate
Childlike
Self-centered
Acts dumb
Little information of intellectual
    nature

Patient's Stream of Thought

Theme songs are usually
    slightly sexualized
Not much concrete information
Hard to develop history
Everything embroidered
Short attention span
Many adventures that scare them
Content relates to old sexual
    material
Still tied to parents
Tells soap opera
Hides what may be disapproved
Hides early material
Tells what a good child he or
    she was
Often tells story of rape never
    told before
Taught sex is no-no
Lots of acting out with little
    sexual pleasure

Histrionic and Dissociative Disorders — page 2

Treatment

Very suggestible

Very responsive—thus, therapist uses influence to get some control

Tells therapist, "you're wonderful, you're brilliant," but doesn't change

Hard to give up fun and games

Clue in to interpretive material

Interesting and cooperative, but hard to keep at work—important to keep
    focus

Don't take away fun and games too fast

Be consistent about being calm and cool

Help to see consequences to behavior

Be supportive but firm

Get into sexual conflict early

Always explore consequences of behavior

Support environmental changes later

Learn to get rid of sexual repression and learn self-approval

Clarify past influences on present

Secondary gains hard to give up

©1994 Michael I. Gold, *The Foundations of Your Private Practice*

Antisocial Personality Disorder
(Psychopathy or Sociopathy)

Pathology

Personality disorder
Symptoms or problems are
  syntonic to patient
Lack of anxiety
Lack of guilt
Asocial
Fairly intractable
Lifelong (before age 15)
No break with reality
Childhood torturing of animals,
  other children

Mood and Affect

Not appropriate
Slight edge
Expectations of therapist too
  high
Therapist may feel manipulated
Seductive
Warm
Responsive
Little anxiety except around
  unpleasant things

General Appearance

Everything OK
May be hostile or negative

Sensorium

Intact—no problem
Doesn't learn from past
  experiences
Information doesn't fit
Overclaiming

Patient's Stream of Thought

How person has been wronged
System is responsible
Takes little responsibility
Conveys how clever and bright
  person is
Lots of lying
Emphasis on ways and means
  to accomplish desires

Treatment Considerations

Long-term commitment
Person uses various kinds of
  relationships to move in slow
  ways
If therapist is trustable, have
  chance
Motivation depends on outside
  pressure
Therapist can be sustainer
Small contracts are useful
Have expectations for person
Contact with significant others
  helps check therapeutic
  distortions
Be careful about promises
Avoid being manipulated
Make ground rules from the
  beginning and stick to them
Align yourself with norms of
  society—there are
  consequences to actions
Focus on impulse control
Reality therapy and responsibility
  emphasis is effective

Notes

Chapter 1

Maslow, Abraham. *Towards a Psychology of Being.* Princeton, NJ: Van Nostrand, Co., 1968.

Chapter 2

Yalom, Irvin D. *Existential Psychotherapy.* New York: Basic Books, 1980.

Chapter 6

Ekstein's lectures were held at the Reiss-Davis Child Study Center in the early 1970s in Los Angeles, California.

Slipp, S. *Object Relations.* New York: Jason Aronson Inc., 1984.

Chapter 10

APA Monitor, August 1990, p. 13.

Chapter 13

Gruen, Arno. *The Betrayal of the Self: The Fear of Autonomy in Men and Women.* New York: Grove Press, 1987.

Chapter 14

Janda, Louis H. and Karin E. Klenke-Hamel. *Human Sexuality.* New York: Van Nostrand, Co., 1980.

Ferris, Sherri. "Selling Your Private Practice: Ten Provocative Questions." *The California Therapist.*

Index

THE FOUNDATIONS OF YOUR PRIVATE PRACTICE
by Michael I. Gold, Ph.D.

Volume One: The Complete Guide to Starting and Developing a Successful Private Practice
Written with Colette McDougall.

This book will help you set up and run a practice as a profitable business. Dr. Gold offers in detail the personal, clinical, and financial aspects of building a successful private practice. The advice and suggestions in this volume will free you as a clinician to devote your creativity and time to your clients—while your practice nearly runs itself.

Contents include: The Ethics of Making Money * The Economics of Private Practice * Selecting Your Location * Setting Up Your Office * Handling Your Practice * Making Your Practice What You Want It to Be * Managing Your Time * Using Your Resources * The Politics of Psychotherapy * Terminating or Selling Your Practice

> "After reviewing these forms, I am convinced they will become the standard of practice in the field."
> — *Richard Marsh, Ph.D., Fellow: American College of Forensic Psychology*
>
> "Dr. Gold's extensive compilation will save hundreds of hours in time and thousands of dollars in consulting fees." — *Ann Spadone Jacobson, Ph.D.*
>
> "This package eliminates the stress of paperwork, from the intake interview through termination."— *Emil Soorani, M.D., Board Certified Psychiatrist/Neurologist*

Volume Two: The Complete Book of Clinical Forms for an Effective Private Practice
Written with Phyllis Galbraith, M.A., and Jean Yingling, M.A., MFCC

This volume is a "private practice in a box": a complete, ready-to-print collection of all the forms necessary to run a practice, developed and tested over 25 years of teaching and clinical work.

The forms, which include a "superbill," are arranged in six groups: Before the Client Arrives * When the Client Arrives * When the Client Is in Session * When There are Special Circumstances * Filling in the Client's Background * Writing Your Reports

The book contains an explanation and filled-in sample of each form. The samples follow the treatment of a clinically normal client and illustrate how the forms aid efficient therapy. There are also sample treatment and evaluation reports.

A full set of blank forms on reproducible cards accompany the volume, and can be personalized for your practice. These forms alone can save thousands of dollars, while costing just one or two hours of billable time.

Volume One ... 192 pages ... Hard cover book ... $29.95
Volume Two ... 184 pages ... Hard cover book ... $74.95
  (Comes with 72-page forms pack)
Clinical Forms only ... 112 pages ... includes sample reports ... $50.00
Volumes One & Two (includes 72-page forms pack) ... $89.95

SUPERBILL: Personalized packs of the "superbill" included with the forms are available in three-part, no-carbon-required (NCR) forms. All the information for one session or a month's worth of sessions is in this one, easy-to-use form. For ordering information, prices, or a sample of the form, call 510-865-5282 or use the order form below.

To order customized overlays for your forms, write to: GMS, P.O. Box 1907, Redondo Beach, CA 90278

—————— SEND ME —————— **ORDER FORM** —————— SHIP TO ——————

FPP1 3/94

Title	Price	Qty	Amount
Sample Superbill	Free	1	Y / N
In California add 7¼% sales tax			
Shipping and handling ($2.50 1st book, $.75 each add'l)			
TOTAL ENCLOSED			

Name

Organization

Street

City/State   Zip

Phone number (for credit card orders)

☐ Check   ☐ Visa   ☐ MC

Card #   Exp date

Signature

Hunter House Inc. Publishers • P.O. Box 2914 • Alameda CA 94501
For quantity discounts call 510/865-5282 or FAX 510/865-4295